THE DREAM CURE

T0340406

THE DREAM CURE

How recalling your dreams can heal your life

THERESA CHEUNG

Thorsons

Harper Thorsons
An imprint of HarperCollins*Publishers*
The News Building
1 London Bridge Street
London SE1 9GF
www.harpercollins.co.uk

HarperCollins*Publishers*
Macken House, 39/40 Mayor Street Upper
Dublin 1, DO1 C9W8, Ireland

First published by Harper Thorsons 2024

1 3 5 7 9 10 8 6 4 2

A catalogue record of this book is available from the British Library.

ISBN 978-0-00-866467-1

Printed and bound in the UK using 100% renewable electricity
at CPI Group (UK) Ltd

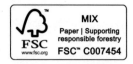

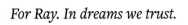

For Ray. In dreams we trust.

'Everything you need to know – all the healing and meaning you need – can be found alive and kicking within your own dreams.'

Theresa Cheung

CONTENTS

Preface: Your Dream Notes   1

Introduction: Messages from your Deep   7

Your Night School   25

Lesson 1: The Stuff of your Dreams   27

Lesson 2: How to Interpret your Dreams   73

Lesson 3: Your Life in your Dreams   120

Lesson 4: Dreaming in your Darkness   203

Lesson 5: Design your Own Dreams   232

Conclusion: You are a Dream   251

Resources   259

Your Dream Cure Journal Templates   260

Index of Dream Themes   264

Suggested Reading, Listening, Watching, Visiting   270

Acknowledgements   274

About the Author   275

YOUR DREAM NOTES

You may not believe it (yet), but your dreams – those fleeting invisible feelings, ideas, stories, symbols and sensations you can sometimes recall on waking – have the power to heal your life. Night after night, they comment on your waking reality and offer you brainstorming creative solutions. They have nothing but your best interests at heart and, most important of all for your personal and spiritual growth, *dreams don't lie.*

The Dream Cure has been written to share with you everything I know (so far) about dream power and how it can dramatically change your life. It was born as a result of my lifetime of dream research, in particular my *Dream Dictionary* which, from its publication in 2004, has been a go-to for decoding dream symbols.

Many of my readers have reached out to me over the years to ask me to offer more practical insight into dream interpretation, and this is what I intend to offer in this book.

To reference the deep wisdom of Confucius, what you hear you forget, what you see you remember, but what you *do* you understand. That's why I designed this book to be as practical as possible, offering you things you can start *doing* immediately to connect to your dream power. I can't wait to show you how you are always talking to yourself in your dreams and how that self-talk is either helping or hindering your progress in waking life. I will also share how dreams can potentially foreshadow your future and how *dreamscaping*, which is the ability to 'incubate' dreams to help solve specific challenges, is a game-changer.

And as a grand finale, when you graduate from your dream cure night school and fully discover just how much dream decoding is healing your life, you will be encouraged to become a dream oracle, dreaming on behalf of others to help them see their own light.

But first let's see what lies ahead for *you*.

BACK TO YOUR NIGHT SCHOOL

Following the introduction, which sets your dream scene, this book is arranged into five 'lessons' to take you on a guided adventure right into the wild heart of your night vision. I will be exploring the most common dream themes and how/why those themes shift through the different stages of life. Virtually no dream theme is left unexplored, and with a handy A to Z index of these themes for easy reference at the back of this book, you'll have at your fingertips all the decoding information you need to become your own dream oracle. And along the way, you will be introduced to simple, highly effective dream-work tools that have the backing of credible research.

My advice is to first read the entire book, because each lesson builds on the momentum created by the previous one.

Then read it again, but this time pause to try out the techniques. Transform each lesson into a self-help session and take a few days to fully savour it. Take all the time you need to personalize your dream work.

A blank notebook or file you can write in, speak to or type in daily to record your dreams and your progress is essential. Keep this journal with you at all times and put it beside your bed before falling asleep. I also suggest you place your copy of *The Dream Cure* on your bedside table as a visual cue. Should you have the digital/audio version, make sure both it and your journal are always readily available, so you can document your dream notes, especially before you go to sleep and on waking.

You'll notice that the introduction, each of the five lessons, plus the conclusion are headed by a *'Night light'* statement which encapsulates the essence of that section. As you read and then work through the techniques suggested in that section, keep referring back to this statement as often as you can, so it has the feel of a recurring dream.

And be sure to take note of, and perhaps even commit to memory, *your dream-work power points (see below)*, which you will be urged to revisit at seminal moments. This refocusing will help reinforce what your unconscious mind must believe to help you get the very best out of your dream work.

Every time you reflect on these power points, notice how, like a dream you can't forget, they constantly yield fresh insights, while at the same time taking you right back to the centre, the heart of your existence, where all meaning is found.

Your dream-work power points

● Dreams don't lie. Your dreams are the deepest and most authentic part of you, revealing the truth beneath the surface, even if that truth hurts.

● Dreams don't happen to you. They are created by and for you.

● How you think and how you feel is how you dream.

● Every dream showcases the power of your present choices and at the same time offers a glimpse of your potential future.

● Dreams reveal your deeply held self-beliefs, and what you believe about yourself is what you attract in waking life.

● Dreams are dreams and you always have the power to change them and therefore your life.

● Nightmares are transformative treasures offering you the opportunity to correct course.

● A dream correctly decoded will raise your energy vibration.

● Your dreams will never ever stop surprising you.

● Fall in love with your dreams and you fall in love with yourself.

⊙ What you dream you are becoming – you are dreaming the future you are attracting with your current mindset – but it's always a potential future and you can always dream another dream.

⊙ Dreams offer you the opportunity to transcend body, logic, reason, space, death and time and see the bigger picture of your life. By so doing, they offer illumination on your waking life, and this is their purpose and true value.

⊙ Your dreams can heal your life.

INTRODUCTION

MESSAGES FROM YOUR DEEP

*Night light: Your dreams are the
deepest and most authentic part of you,
the place where everything begins
and never ends.*

Dreams are the centre of your existence. They are unseen messages from the depths of your heart, aka your unconscious. They tell you what your waking intuition has noticed because it is important for your personal growth, but your ego is blocking from your conscious awareness.

Every single night your dreams take you beyond time and space on a fantastic voyage of infinite self-discovery. Once you can get past their mystery and discover for yourself just how effortless it is to understand and work with them, they can help you get answers, find meaning, generate ideas, let go of fears, reduce stress, attract success, glimpse your future and so much more.

In essence, your dreams are your secret superpower, forever striving to heal and empower you from the inside out. They are your inner therapist and counsellor. After reading this book, I hope you will never again allow their priceless wisdom to slip away.

MY DREAM ADVENTURE

I have little doubt that dream decoding can heal my life in every way possible. I know that understanding my dreams is understanding the depths of myself. I know they shine a night light on my current mindset and what it is attracting into my reality. I know they can illuminate all areas of my life. I know that working with them constantly delights and surprises me and changes absolutely everything. However, it wasn't always this way.

To provide context, let me briefly share the story of my dream life so far...

From an early age I was encouraged to ponder and relish the mystery and wisdom of my vivid dreams. I would eagerly debate their meaning every morning with my Spiritualist family. I hoped to continue that debate when I went to study for my degree at King's College, Cambridge University, but quickly found that academic study of dreams was deemed unscientific.

So, when I left university, I researched dreams independently and in 2004 I was offered the opportunity to write *The Dream Dictionary from A to Z*. It's still in print today. I have had countless messages from readers over the years asking for help with interpreting their dreams. And what they are hoping for isn't general interpretation, but bespoke insight, personal to them.

This never amazes me, as humans have always looked to their dreams for meaning. In centuries past, shamans, oracles, priests and other intuitive guides were sought out for their interpretations. Then the position of dream decoder fell to psychiatrists and therapists, each with their own theories on dream meanings, but the people who write to me aren't typically in need of therapy. They are simply eager to learn what *their* dreams are trying to tell *them*.

I studied every school of dream interpretation in depth and learned much of immense value, but over time I came to the conclusion that in most cases the best person to interpret a dream isn't a therapist or dream 'expert', but the dreamer themselves. I also came to the conclusion that as we all dream, we can all discover how to interpret our own dreams and use their insight to guide our waking lives. So, in hindsight, this book was always a dream waiting to be written.

But it simply wouldn't have been possible for me to write it until now. Although dreams have always enchanted me, it is only in the last few years that I have fully woken up to and lived and breathed their healing power.

Prior to that, I saw them as sacred gifts, a nightly reassurance that there is more to life than meets the eye. And my belief in dreams as spontaneous spiritual revelations was reflected back to me. Indeed, on one occasion I believe a dream saved my life. I was in my early thirties at the time and driving to a busy junction, fully intending to turn left. But then a memory of the previous night's dream of my departed mother telling me to take the right path flashed into my mind. I instinctively obeyed and later found out that if I had turned left, I would have almost certainly been involved in a fatal vehicle pile-up.

As miraculous as this 'dream saved my life' experience was, and as much as it filled me with a renewed passion for promoting dream power, it was just the tip of the nocturnal iceberg. I still had a great deal to learn about the countless ways dreaming could truly save my life.

FROM GRIEF TO GROWTH

Around seven years ago, the foundations of my life were rocked by a series of traumatic personal losses and professional mishaps. Every aspect of my life felt misaligned, the deepest pain being that my partner of twenty-five years suffered an irreversible brain injury with accompanying memory loss, casting me wholly unprepared into the demanding role of carer.

I felt frightened, vulnerable and alone, grieving the gradual loss of my partner's identity. I didn't know if I had the strength to cope with the rapidly changing circumstances of my life. Despair wasn't an entirely new experience for me. I had been deep down there before in my late teens and early adult life, but escaped its clutches as I poured my heart and soul into raising my two children and writing a series of books about dreams and other metaphysical subjects. However, here it was right back again – that familiar darkness, my unwelcome old friend.

I tried all the advised self-help. Visited my GP. I meditated. Practised positive rituals and went for long, brisk walks. I reached out for help, for advice from loved ones, therapists and support groups and forums. I journalled. I prayed. I cried as often as I needed to. I attended vibration-raising webinars and reread seminal spiritual books and quotes. I tried everything. Some things helped for a while. Nothing stuck.

After months of struggling to find my light, I fell into bed one particularly cold winter's evening, feeling broken, empty. Nothing I was absorbing seemed to be giving me the vibrational shift I urgently needed. Even my normally sharp dream recall had vanished. The words 'Help me' looped in my mind as I drifted into a heavy sleep.

On waking the next morning, a carnival of intensely clear dream memories greeted me. I instinctively reached for my dream journal to write them down, and as I did, more and more bizarre sensations, stories, symbols, thoughts, sounds and feelings flooded in. My hands couldn't keep up with the words I needed to record. Never in my life had I experienced dream overcrowding like this before.

Sharing the sensations swirling in my mind that morning would fill the pages of this book, so I will restrain myself. Although dream sharing is something you may want to consider, as it boosts empathy, one thing I have learned is that it isn't a helpful starting-point. This is because the power of dream work lies in your own *direct, personal experience* and the relationship you create with your own dreams. You need to understand and experience their power *first*, before sharing them with others and being bombarded with their dreams in turn. Information is not knowledge. The only source of knowledge is experience.

So, I've resisted the temptation to punctuate this book with my dreams or, as fascinating as they are, the dreams sent to me by my readers. From start to finish I want this book to be about *you* – and what you can discover from your own priceless dreams.

However, to return briefly to my morning of 1,000 dreams, the message I want to share here is although they didn't immediately make any sense at all, they brought a mighty and much-needed shift towards self-reflection and inner empowerment. I wrote down as many as I could recall, and some of the visions I recorded would later translate into future books, but the greatest gift these symbols from my deep gave me was the reassurance that I wasn't alone, or empty. My inner world was calling my name. It was filled with surprises and hope. The help I was seeking wasn't out there. It was alive and kicking within.

I needed to trust as never before in my own inner space, and see my challenges as opportunities for spectacular growth and my newfound role as carer as a privilege I had been chosen for. I needed to turn my problems into purpose and get excited about the new horizons they signalled. In the midst of my winter, my own dreams were showing me there was an invincible summer within me.

Although I carried on doing all the practical self-help advised, instead of hoping for a miracle to happen externally, every night before falling asleep I would ask my dreaming mind to show itself. Waking up with dreams to ponder brought me tremendous resilience and the realization that I was going to cope. I had my own back.

I fully understood as never before that my dreams reflected my relationship with myself and that relationship was creating my waking life. And this newfound reconnection to my own depths gave me the courage to experiment with a range of techniques that could influence the contents of my dreams. I figured if I could change my dreams, I could change my unconscious negative beliefs and what they were manifesting. I could transform ingrained feelings of helplessness into feelings of empowerment.

Time and time again since then my night visions have picked me up when I have fallen down. They have also helped me – and continue to help me – choose and attract the life, the future, of my dreams.

Today, I feel stronger, wiser and more positive than ever. My professional life is on track and, most importantly, my partner and family are content, making the best of every precious day. I can honestly say I have dream work to thank for that healing transformation.

I still believe dreams are sacred gifts. (That's why I treat every dream that is shared with me with the deepest respect, because whenever you share your dreams, you may not realize it, but what you are revealing is a piece of your soul.) However, my essential shift in perspective came from knowing my dreams didn't just happen *to* me. Dreams are created *by* and happen *for* me to help me learn, grow and return to wholeness from the inside out. Just as they are for you.

DREAM POWER

After experiencing how much my dreams helped me not just survive but thrive during a time of personal crisis, I revisited all my previous dream research and decided it was high time to place dream power centre-stage.

I started to write, teach and speak about dreams more and more and, as like seeks like, more and more requests for my dream expertise steadily came in. Some people were mystified by my newfound focus. I lost count of the number of times I heard, 'But it's just a dream,' which made it crystal clear to me that most people had absolutely no idea that their 'crazy' dreaming mind was a source of brilliant illumination. And those who were intrigued only had a superficial understanding of dream work; that's why so many misunderstandings linger on and the full potential of dreaming as a personal growth tool is still not being realized.

It became my calling to educate as many people as I could about the healing potential of their own dreams, to help others understand that the relationship you have with your dreams can set the tone for what you think, feel, do and ultimately attract into your life. Changing your dreams, rather than your thoughts, is the real secret of manifestation, because your dreams showcase the unconscious limiting beliefs that you don't always know that you have, but repeatedly stop you in your tracks.

A dream is a wish your heart makes when you're fast asleep. Disney got that right. But a dream is more than a wish. It is also a problem-solver, a creativity hack, a stressbuster, an entertainer, a holistic healer. It is also a dynamic manifesting tool, because you really can positively influence the contents of your dreams. And whenever shifts happen at this deep unconscious level, things start to shift in your conscious life.

I continue to defer to my dreams, and on days when my recall is poor, I know that this in itself is a subtle message from my dreaming mind. It is a sign that I may be falling into the trap of seeking validation from externals again, from other people and things, rather than my own inner compass. It's a signal I need to spend more of my waking hours looking within and reflecting deeply on what my values are.

Today, simply thinking about the potential of my dreams to empower me from the inside out never fails to fill me with gratitude, anticipation and a sense of infinite possibility. It signals to me that whatever challenges life throws at me, there is always something strong, something better and something infinitely creative pushing right back. There is always another dream to pull me forward and remind me of my own inner power. To remind me that the most important relationship of all is the one I have with myself.

SACRED SCIENCE AND ART

In recent years, I've seen a surge of interest in dreams and their meaning. This gathered pace during the pandemic with the well-reported lockdown dream phenomenon.

During the lockdowns, many people felt isolated and suffered great personal loss, but woke up to vivid dream recall. Altered sleep patterns, combined with the removal of external distractions, gave dreams the space they needed to surface and remind people of their neglected inner world.

There was an unprecedented spike in dream recall, which was reported globally for the first time thanks to the prevalence of social media use and people sharing their dreams with one another. This led to a wealth of much-needed and ongoing research, but although this spirit of investigation has its positives for many people, the amount of new information currently coming out is overwhelming. It can be hard to know where to start, so I have pored over this research and collated it into five simple lessons for your personal growth.

Before you dive in, it is important to point out that although dream work is currently peaking in popularity, it is not a New Age trend or fad. People have been interpreting their dreams since time immemorial, with perhaps the earliest evidence of dream interpretation being found in ancient Mesopotamian and Egyptian papyri and clay tablets.

Dream work was regarded as a sacred art and science in all ancient civilizations. It has always been and remains a potent self-help tool. It now has the added benefit of being backed by credible research, making it an accessible and an exciting crossroads where science and spirit can happily converge.

DREAM ON IT

Yes, dreams are strange and may often feel utterly incomprehensible, but as you will learn in the pages that follow, there is always method in their madness. Once you learn this method, you'll find that your dreams are your ultimate reality check. They are your most devoted friend, the one who stands by you regardless, refreshingly honest and always there for you.

The pressures of daily life can sometimes be too much to resolve when you are awake. The answers, leaps of faith and creative connections you need can often only be found when your logical mind is sleeping and your intuition is unleashed in your dreams.

You are always your own best adviser, but sometimes it takes a whole lot of self-awareness and self-belief to get the message through. Working with your dreams can fast-track you to that game-changing self-awareness and trust, especially when other self-help tools have failed.

The simple truth is that your greatest inspirations, Eureka moments, personal realizations and self-healing leaps don't always happen when you are in a state of flow, or when you're meditating, or even when you're in the shower. They happen all the time in your dreams. I'm sure at some point in your life you have been told to 'sleep on it', but what this really means is 'dream on it'.

The best is always yet to come when you fall asleep, and waking up with dream recall is an everyday miracle that can always be relied upon to raise your vibration. And your awareness.

Understanding the wisdom of your dreams can heal your life.

WHAT YOUR DREAMS WANT YOU TO KNOW

If your dreaming mind could talk to you right now in words rather than feelings and symbols, here are some fragments it would want you to imprint on your heart.

Your dreams want a committed long-term relationship with you

Your dreams long to be recalled, noticed and taken seriously by you. They want to enter into a full-blown relationship with you. Whenever you ignore or dismiss them, they feel directionless, purposeless, invisible, unloved and alone.

And your dreams don't just want a one-night stand! They want a long-term commitment. It frustrates them when you are all in for one dream and then forget about them the next night. Every night they appear like a long-running TV series you need to tune into again and again for the next thrilling instalment of yourself. They are in this with you forever!

The more you love them, the more they will reward you

When it comes to dreams, as with anything in life, the more you put in, the more you get out. If you cherish all your dreams and make even the seemingly trivial and mundane ones feel special, in return they will offer you ever-increasing revelations.

What you dream is what you attract

Your dreams symbolically reflect to you your current relationship with yourself. This is important, because what you think and feel about yourself is the reality you are likely to create and attract in waking life. In this way, every dream reminds you that you and only you choose what you feel, think and do. You are the creator of both your reality and the dreams powering it.

The power is always within you

Every time you give your power away to the expectations of others or your happiness and self-worth rest on material outcomes, whether those be money, popularity or status, your dreams will send you a clear and present warning, either through an anxiety-themed dream or through lack of dream recall, that you are heading in the wrong direction.

Your dreams love solving puzzles

Every dream you recall is sharing with you a potential solution to your waking challenges. Whatever the challenge, your dreams will get to work on your behalf, offering brainstorming solutions. Nothing is off-limits. All you need to do is trust them.

What you choose to believe and therefore dream about is what becomes true for you

Your dreaming mind accepts what you choose to think and believe as truth (even if that is an unconscious choice) and reveals that truth clearly to you. If you choose to believe you are unlovable, this is what you will see in both your dreams and in your life. Knowing this reminds you that your thoughts and dreams are unlimited and intertwined. Choose to incubate different dreams and this will impact your thoughts. Choose different thoughts and this will influence your dreamscape.

Your dreams don't judge or belittle you

Your dreams accept you for who you are. Their intention is never to judge, criticize or belittle. They understand that you are a work in progress and on an endless learning curve. They understand that many of your damaging beliefs are not your own – they have been imposed on you since you were a child, by parents, teachers, friends, colleagues, society, your job and others. Your dreams simply want you to become aware of these self-limiting beliefs so that you can let those limitations go and rediscover your own identity.

The fact you are reading this book is a sign that you are ready to know the truth about yourself and to empower your life from the inside out. Your dreaming mind is noticing and loudly applauding you!

Your dreams show you that what you feel about other people is within you

Recognizing that the people who appear in your dreams are often symbolic representations of your own inner fears or aspects of yourself you need to face or embody reminds you yet again that nobody in your waking life has any power over you unless you give it to them.

Every dream you have is trying to encourage you to take back your own power.

They remind you that your power is always in the *now*

Your dreams and waking life are interconnected. You don't stop being you when you dream, you just enter a different state of consciousness. Your dreams are fiercely current, always problem-solving your present reality and the implications this creates for your potential future.

And contrary to what you may believe, dreaming of your past isn't about the past, it's always about what's going on for you now. Your dreaming mind is simply using symbols from your past to alert you to similar patterns surfacing in your present.

How you think is how you dream

Your dreams reflect your thoughts and feelings about yourself. Often you aren't fully aware of limiting mindsets in your waking life, but you can see them clearly in your dreams.

This point is so important that your dreaming mind never tires of restating it, often through recurring dream themes. Your dreams reveal, in a symbolic vision, the unconscious beliefs that create your thoughts. They shine light on the deepest part of you, offering you an opportunity to become aware, understand and then change unconscious limitations and therefore the present they are creating and the future they are attracting.

Not recalling your dreams is another way they speak to you

Unless there are medical reasons or you suffer from a sleep disorder (and if that is the case, talk to your GP as soon as you can), if your dream recall is consistently poor, your dreaming mind wants you to restore balance in your waking life.

Inner peace comes when there is a balance between the external and the internal, the logical and the intuitive. If you can't recall your dreams, there may be too much focus on your waking life, on the material 'stuff' or on what is happening outside you. You need to find balance by consciously connecting to your inner world through journalling, daydreaming, listening to music, reading fiction and poetry, drawing, dancing, spending time in nature or simply reflecting on the mystery of life.

The more creative and empowering your dreams, the more your self-love will grow

Self-love is the journey of all our lives. Dream work is the ideal place to start if you, like many people, struggle to think positively about yourself, however many affirmations you do. If you don't believe in or love yourself, it makes it harder for others to do so, because like attracts like. Understanding the healing magic of your dreams and approaching them with an earnest desire to understand them better can help you start to fall in love with yourself from the inside out. And when that happens, you become an unstoppable force.

Your dreams help you let go

Your dreams want you to know that letting go isn't a loss. It can feel beautiful, like watching the glorious colours of leaves falling from autumn trees. Releasing but not forgetting the past – because forgetting means you are destined to repeat it – is how you learn and grow.

Sometimes letting go is simply forgiving. Not forgetting, but forgiving. Often the thing you find the hardest to face and forgive in yourself and others appears as the dominant recurring theme of your dreams, because it's the thing you most need to let go of.

Your dreams want many things for you, but most of all they long for you to release yourself from what holds you back so you can learn and grow.

Your waking reality is a mirror of your inner world

People tend to treat you in waking life the way you treat your-self, and night after night your dreams remind you of that life hack. When you fully understand this, your dreams will shift to higher and more creative levels.

You are more than your body and mind

Whatever happens in your waking life, within you there is something deeply mysterious and creative that can rise above and be untouchable. This is the deepest part of yourself that isn't defined by the material, your body or even your mind. It is the most authentic part of you, revealed to you night after night in your dreams – your soul, for want of a better word.

Dreams want you to love yourself just the way you are

Your dreaming mind wants you to know that when you under-stand, love and accept yourself in the present moment, just the way you are, then your waking life will heal. It wants you to replace self-reproach with self-compassion, because then you can move away from those repetitive dreams of falling, drowning and silent screams to a whole new multiverse of flying, dancing, space and other infinitely expansive dream potentials.

Ah, with this newfound knowledge fresh from this conversation with your night vision, what dreams for you, dear reader, may come!

ARE YOU READY TO UNLOCK YOUR DREAM DOOR?

Now you have heard the clear and present voice of your dreams calling out to you, the scene is set. Time now for the night light to shine directly on you and your always astonishing dreams.

Are *you* ready to continue this deep conversation with your dreams and begin the first lesson of your night school?

Are you ready to unlock the door to your dreams, engage with the illuminating power of your night vision and allow it to do what it does best – heal your life?

YOUR NIGHT SCHOOL

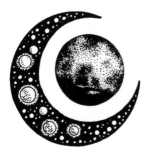

Night is the parent of all thoughts and feelings and the deeply held dreams that power them...

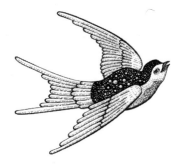

THE STUFF OF YOUR DREAMS

Night light: Dream work is proactive self-care, an act of self-respect. To prioritize your dream recall is to prioritize yourself.

Waking up in the middle of the night, when darkness and mystery surround you, can give the sensation of floating in space.

Next time you have an unscheduled night waking, stay calm, breathe deeply, settle down, close your eyes, and as you drift back to sleep, focus gently on the canvas shimmering behind your eyes. You may see spots of light, shapes and patterns dancing there like shooting stars.

That's your night vision offering a sneak preview of coming attractions, reminding you that your infinite inner space, rather than your outer space, is the place to boldly go and seek out new horizons. It's gently enticing you to leap beyond time and space and return to the whirlpool of mystery and infinite possibility that is the land of dreams.

But what are dreams?

DREAM, DREAM, DREAM

Dreams are a universal human experience that can be described as a state of consciousness characterized by sensory, cognitive and emotional occurrences during sleep.

Standard dictionary definition

While you are sleeping, your dreaming mind orchestrates a series of images and sensations uniquely designed to unleash your intuition and offer you new perspectives that can guide you towards finding meaning and healing from the inside out.

Waking up to the power of your dreams to guide you can be compared to the frog in the well metaphor. The frog believes that the well (waking life and the material world) is the only reality, not realizing that an ocean of adventure (dreams and what is unseen) could be theirs if only they took a giant leap of faith.

Dream images and sensations are symbolic recreations of things your unconscious or intuition has noticed during the day because they are important for your personal growth, but your waking mind has either not noticed them or dismissed them because they seem illogical. However, when you fall asleep, material distractions and logic vanish, offering your intuition an opportunity to take centre-stage and speak to you about what really matters.

In essence, to quote from the epic 1965 science-fiction novel and 2021 blockbuster movie *Dune*, 'Dreams are messages from your deep.'

When you dream, you enter the alternate reality of your unconscious and the hidden treasures of your own deep. Nothing is impossible, except reason. Impossible belongs to the waking world. In dreams, 'impossible' translates to 'I'm possible'. You can transcend space and time. You can become anyone. You can go anywhere and do anything.

Despite nothing being out of bounds, sometimes dreams can recreate what feels very familiar to you from your waking life. But dreams that feel exceedingly ordinary can still offer deep insight. There is no such thing as a meaningless dream. Everyone has at some point in their life had the experience of waking up with a dream on their mind that feels so real it is impossible to forget. And in that surreal moment, you ponder what dreams are and what on Earth they mean.

WHY DREAM?

There are a number of credible theories about this and a great deal of research has been done, but as yet there is no definite explanation. Despite the best efforts of scientists to define them, much like the rest of the human brain or the nature of consciousness itself, dreams remain an enticing enigma.

The only majority opinion is that we all dream at least five or six times every night – dreams illustrate what unites rather than divides humanity. Brain scans show that those who say they don't dream do. They just don't remember their dreams.

The study and science of dreams is called *oneirology*. There is so much yet to learn, but the more we learn about dreams – what they are, why we have them, what they mean – the more we learn about who we are, why we are here and what the meaning of our mysterious lives might be.

The long-held notion that dreams are simply random and nonsensical firings of the brain persists, but in recent years there has been a growing acknowledgement among scientists that dreams do have a role to play in holistic well-being. Indeed, extreme anxiety occurs if subjects are deprived of REM sleep – the rapid eye movement stage when most, but not all, dreaming occurs. This is a promising sign that, although we don't really know why, dreaming is good for us.

In ancient times it was thought that dreams were from another dimension. Some continue to believe this, but the majority of dream experts, myself included, now believe that dreams come from our unconscious – that they are thoughts, feelings and impulses that have not been noticed or expressed in waking life. In this way, dreams are like an inner therapist, allowing the dreamer to brainstorm connections, learn about what matters to them and face and deal with unresolved feelings and thoughts to achieve inner peace.

In addition to being highly cathartic and therapeutic, dreams offer a nightly simulation experience where you can safely rehearse skills or 'act out' worst-case scenarios so you are better prepared to cope in your waking life. They also help you make sense of all the information you encounter in your day, and are therefore vital for brain health, memory consolidation and learning.

Not to mention dreams aid problem-solving and ignite serious creativity. If you have ever woken up in the morning with illumination, chances are it has been because a dream has been working silently behind the scenes to inspire you. Indeed, visions in dreams have been responsible for world-changing theories, inventions and works of art. Many of us don't consider ourselves visionary in waking life, but dreams show that when we fall asleep, we are true visionaries.

In a nutshell, there are many 'whys' rather than one single 'why' we dream, and all of them work synergistically, the uniting factor being that an active dream life is connected to an active brain and holistic well-being. Scientists, most notably Matthew Walker, professor of psychology and neuroscience at the University of California, Berkeley, and numerous peer-reviewed studies are rapidly coming to the conclusion that dreaming could be as important for our heath as food, drink and the air we breathe. Indeed, according to a 2017 review about dreaming published in the *Annals* of the New York Academy of Sciences, lack of REM (dreaming) sleep, rather than poor sleep, is responsible for many emotional and health problems.

THE SLEEPING BRAIN

To understand dreams better, scientists study the place of their origin – the brain – and what parts of the brain remain 'awake' when a person falls asleep.

When you are sleeping, your limbic or emotional, intuitive brain centres become more active than the logical, rational brain centres. This makes sense, as when you wake up, it is the feelings of your dream that you are likely to recall first, rather than the scenarios. The absence of waking logic and reason allows the suspension of disbelief and explains why in the dream state the bizarre feels normal and you can make creative connections your waking logic wouldn't allow you to even contemplate.

Intriguingly, research also indicates that during REM sleep, noradrenaline, a fight-or-flight hormone similar to adrenaline, is absent. In the other sleep stages and the waking state, it is present. This is significant because with no noradrenaline and the limbic parts of the brain active, the dreaming mind can conjure up scenarios and process information in a way that feels both natural and stress-free. In the safety of a dream, the brain can process trauma without the risk of emotional pain.

As well as differences between the dreaming and waking brain, scientists also look for similarities. One of those is the brain activity involved in facial recognition. It seems that dreaming of a face activates the same part of the brain as recognizing a face when you are awake.

All this research into the dreaming brain and how it differs from or compares to the waking brain is exciting, because it helps us understand the nature of consciousness better. It also suggests that while dreams are certainly influenced by waking reality, they aren't entirely created by it. Something happens in the dreaming state that can't yet be explained.

YOU SLEEP TO DREAM

In addition to studying the dreaming brain, scientists also study the place where dreams begin – sleep.

Guess what? In much the same way that they don't really know why we dream, they don't really know why we sleep either. They have many theories about the whys of sleep, but the only thing they can agree on is that sleep is essential for survival. If we are completely sleep-deprived, death will follow.

You probably think that you sleep because you need to rest and rejuvenate, and while rejuvenation does happen on a physical level when you sleep, rest doesn't. Your body remains active while you sleep, with twitching movements, and your brain, of course, remains active in the dreaming state.

Given the proven holistic healing benefits of dreaming, in my humble opinion the reason we sleep is because we urgently need to dream.

STEPPING INTO YOUR DREAMS

Most dreams occur in the REM (rapid eye movement) stage of sleep, where your eyes dart around following your dreams. However, dreams can also happen in the deeper stages of sleep, although they tend to be less vivid and harder to recall.

There are five stages of sleep, which repeat around four or five times for every eight hours of sleep. Each is characterized by a change in brain waves, the neural function or electrical activity in the brain.

In the first stage of sleep, as you start to doze off, your body temperature drops slightly and breathing and heart rate slow down. Alpha and theta brain waves characterize this state. It is often called the hypnagogic state. You are not yet unconscious and dreaming, but getting there, and may experience images behind your eyes. This sleep stage has creative potential and we will return to it later in this book. (On waking, your state is similar, but called the hypnopompic state.)

The second and third stages of sleep continue the falling asleep process, with your breathing and pulse slowing down further. You gradually lose awareness of externals and the alpha and theta brain waves are replaced by slow delta ones. In the fourth, deep sleep stage, delta brain waves are dominant and there is minimal bodily activity.

The fifth stage of sleep is REM, and during this lighter sleep stage the characteristic brain waves are a mixture of alpha and theta, which is fairly similar to the waking state. Breathing and heart rate are more rapid and the eyes move rapidly behind closed lids. Dreams typically happen when you are in the REM stage and your brain activity is similar to when you are awake. If you wake up immediately after an REM cycle, you are more likely to recall a dream than if you wake after the other stages of sleep.

If you wake too rapidly during this stage, you may feel unable to move, because your body has been temporarily relaxed to stop you acting out your dreams. This is 'sleep paralysis' and most of us aren't aware it happens naturally every time we fall asleep.

A BRIEF HISTORY OF DREAM WORK

Before you begin your night school in earnest, it is important to recognize that dream work is not a New Age trend. It is innate. You are walking in ancient footsteps.

From our very first sleeps on this Earth, dreams have enchanted us. Some ancient cultures believed them to be divine downloads and a door to the afterlife, others regarded them as prophecies. To this day, indigenous shamanic cultures have a deep respect for the dream world.

Stone Age cave art suggests an awareness of dreams and their meanings. Dream interpretations have been found etched onto Mesopotamian clay tablets dating back to 5000 BCE. Perhaps the earliest dream dictionary was created around 1220 BCE in Thebes, Egypt. It is called the papyrus Chester Beatty 3 and the British Museum is its home. This artefact offers contrary prophetic dream analysis in that negative symbols have a positive interpretation and positive symbols have a negative interpretation. For example, death in a dream suggests long life. Sexual arousal suggests victory for enemies.

The auspicious/inauspicious power of dreams remained largely unquestioned until the time of the ancient Greeks, when Plato (427–348 BCE) and his pupil Aristotle (384–322 BCE) suggested that dreams were more likely to be related to the dreamer's feelings and mindset.

The most notable person to popularize dream interpretation is thought to be a Roman called Artemidorus (138–180 CE), who lived in Greek Asia Minor. Ahead of his time, he suggested that although dream symbols had common interpretations, the personal association the dreamer had with the symbol, as well as the conditions of their waking life, had to be taken into account.

From the Middle Ages onwards, dream interpretation was swiftly sidelined and repressed by the Church in particular. The idea that dreams were either meaningless or dangerous to meddle with continued for several hundred years until the early nineteenth century, with the dawn of the Romantic movement and its spirited rebellion against the dominance of reason.

The Romantics championed individual creativity, setting the scene for the rediscovery of dream work. Dream interpretation was considered worthy again and the publication of books such as *The Royal Book of Dreams* by Robert Cross Smith in 1830 paved the way for the popular revival of dream work that was cemented by the godfathers of modern dream interpretation: Sigmund Freud (1856–1939) and Carl Jung (1875–1961).

Freud and Jung pioneered the concept that dreams were symbolic representations of the dreamer's unconscious feelings and interpreting those symbols could offer considerable illumination to the dreamer's waking life.

Other notable dream leaders included Alfred Alder (1870–1937), who proposed that dreams were largely wish-fulfilment, and Fritz Perls (1893–1970), who suggested that dream symbols pointed to aspects of the personality not being expressed.

These seminal dream approaches all played their part in ensuring that dream interpretation is now a credible personal growth tool. There continues to be differences of opinion among modern dream experts on the best way to understand and work with dreams. But the general consensus is that dreams are an inner guidance system offering invaluable insights from the unconscious for personal growth and healing.

MORE THAN THAT

So, dream work is potent self-help therapy, but it is so much more than that. It can also help you attract success and happiness into your life. I believe it is the most frequently neglected manifesting tool.

Did you know that experiencing in the dream state what you want to happen in your waking life is a sign you are close to manifesting it? At a deep unconscious level, you believe it is possible and there is tremendous power in belief.

Everything is energy, including the stars, the sky, the oceans, you, your thoughts and your feelings. And like attracts like. What you believe about yourself and your life is what you tend to attract. In your dreams, you get an intimate presentation of your unconscious beliefs – beliefs that you may not be aware of or willing to admit to when you are awake. Therein lies the real power of dreams. They showcase beliefs that aren't helping you, offering you an opportunity to consciously choose more empowering beliefs when you are awake.

Sadly, the majority of dreams tend to be anxiety related, because so many of us, deep down, don't truly believe in ourselves. But there are things you can do to influence the contents of your dreams so your night vision is on your side, attracting success rather than repelling it.

That's why later in this night school you'll learn not just how to recall and understand your dreams and therefore yourself better, but also how to mould your dreams so they can get to work on your behalf, challenging unconscious abundance blocks so you can open the door and let happiness in.

Dreaming of what you want is actually a sign you believe it is possible for you to have it, and when you have that level of belief in yourself, you are close to manifesting it, bringing a whole new world of meaning to that cliché: 'If you can dream it, you can do it.' Like many clichés, it is true.

So, are you ready to dream bigger and better? High time to enter the temple of your dreams.

THE TEMPLE OF YOUR DREAMS

YOUR SAFE PLACE TO DREAM

To risk stating the obvious, the best place to begin your big dream-work adventure is in your bedroom. If your sleeping environment isn't optimizing your chances of a good night's sleep, physical and mental fatigue will block your chances of dream recall. Your bedroom needs to be associated with security and relaxation, both physical and mental. It is your sanctuary, your dream temple.

Here are some practical things you need to put into place immediately to boost both your quality of sleep and your dream recall:

- Declutter your bedroom, and that includes your wardrobe, drawers and the space under the bed. You don't need to be a *feng shui* or tidying-up expert to know that clutter can escalate stress.

⚇ Remove any work-related items and electrical items. If you must charge your phone in your bedroom, place it as far away from your bed as you can, and keep it on silent when you go to sleep, except for emergency calls.

⚇ Is the paintwork or wallpaper in your bedroom dreamy? I suggest calming blue or purple or skin-tone colours. Sometimes just the addition of an inspiring picture is enough to set the scene. My perfect dream nourishment is my poster of Salvador Dalí's 'Persistence of Memory'.

⚇ The perfect sleeping temperature is cooler than you may think at around 15–19 degrees C (60–67 degrees F). Your body needs to cool down before you drift off to sleep and overheating is a common cause of poor sleep hygiene, as is too much light. Invest in some blackout blinds if you have to. Noise should also be kept to a minimum.

TIMING

Sleep experts agree that going to sleep before midnight and getting around eight hours of sleep a night is optimum. Having said that, everyone is unique, and teenagers and people with medical conditions may need considerably more sleep. If you wake up feeling rested and alert, chances are you got a good night's sleep.

You can invest in apps or watches that track your sleeping habits, with some of them telling you how much REM sleep you got. In my experience, although these can be helpful in getting you interested in your sleep cycles, in the long term they can add to stress and self-reproach. The last thing you need when you wake up feeling depleted is a reminder of that fact beeping on your phone.

If you wake up feeling tired, the most likely reason for it is that you have sleep debt. The best way to fix that is not to stare at data, but to get enough daylight during the day, ensure your bedroom is conducive to sleep and go to bed an hour or half an hour before you normally do. A lie-in is a tempting idea, but this can be very confusing for your body clock, giving you the jet-lag without the holiday.

Although your dreams love wild spontaneity, your body loves routine. Give it a regular 'going to sleep' time, ideally before midnight, and as often as you can, aim to wake up around the same time each morning.

Ditch the alarm clock

You may think your alarm clock is your friend. It allows you to fall asleep without having to worry about waking up in time for work or whatever your day ahead holds for you. Sorry to break it to you, but your alarm clock is your foe. It isn't just bad for you physically, with some experts saying that waking up to the shocking sound of an alarm clock is traumatic for your body and heart, but it isn't good news for your mind and dream recall either, for the simple reason that it shocks you into waking reality far too quickly. Dreams, coming as they do from your invisible depths, struggle to make their presence felt, and recall will be poor.

If you can train yourself to wake up naturally, your health will benefit. And if you can programme yourself to wake up naturally, there's no reason why you can't programme yourself to recall your dreams.

To wake naturally, before you go to sleep, set the intention to wake up at a certain time. And then, when you wake up naturally at the agreed time, get up. Keep setting the intention to wake up naturally every night and in a few weeks it will become routine.

If you are worried you might oversleep, the best advice is to set the intention to wake up five minutes *before* your alarm goes off, so if for some reason you don't wake up naturally, you still have the alarm as a back-up. And make sure your alarm isn't a ring-tone but nature sounds, such as birds singing or cows mooing, or better still, use an alarm that vibrates gently on your wrist.

Now you have your dream temple in order, let's look at some of the other challenges to dream work that you might encounter.

CHALLENGES TO DREAM WORK

POOR DREAM RECALL

The most obvious challenge to dream work is not recalling your dreams. This doesn't mean you don't dream, because brain scans show we all dream at least five or six times each night. When you were a child and suspending disbelief came naturally, you probably had no problem recalling your dreams, but since then you may have got into the habit of just getting up and rushing into your day. This will have knocked the confidence of your dreaming mind. Like an old friend who keeps texting you and never receives a reply, sooner or later your dreaming mind will learn to become silent. So, you need to start doing all you can to reassure it that you are there for it and want a dialogue with it.

Fortunately, in the great majority of cases, with three simple changes your dream memory will return.

Change your perspective

The first change is to your perspective. One of the biggest reasons you may struggle to recall your dreams is that you haven't been taking them seriously until now. Where your mindset is during the day is what is reflected back at you in your dreams. I hope reading this book will change that perspective forever. As often as you can during the day, think about the potential of your dreams to heal your life and how exciting this is.

Make some power moves

The second change is to follow through that change in perspective with these quick-fix dream-recall power moves:

- Before you go to bed at night, place your dream journal and pen or voice recorder beside your bed, or within easy reach, as a visual cue to record your dreams on waking. If you need a torch, make sure that is there too.

- Set the intention to dream before you fall asleep. Simply tell yourself (whisper it out loud) as you drift off to sleep that you are going to recall your dreams on waking.

On waking, stay still for a couple of minutes with your eyes closed. Avoid getting up right away. You want to stay close to your dream physically, and any movement, even blinking, will redirect your focus from the unconscious to the conscious waking state.

If no images appear, just let your mind wander or recall a previous night's dream, as often this will trigger a memory.

Notice areas of tension in your body, as dream memories may be stored there.

Notice how you feel, as the language of dreams is emotion.

When memories surface (and they will), write them down or record them immediately. Writing is advised, as it is more calming, but do whatever works best for you. Don't go to the bathroom or do anything else, unless you absolutely have to, because if you do, those dream memories will vanish, however certain you are that you can retain them.

Prep during the day

The third, and perhaps most important, change is to do things during the day and before sleeping that will increase your chances of dream recall:

Make sure you eat healthily and especially get your B vitamins, in particular vitamin B6, which has been shown to boost dream recall. It's found in bananas, eggs, nuts and wholegrains, and it's best to get it that way rather than as a supplement. If you want to take a supplement, be sure to consult your doctor or a medical professional first.

- Your sleep schedule is dictated by your circadian rhythm, which is the daily cycle of when you feel awake and when you feel sleepy. Your circadian rhythm is governed by cycles of light and darkness, both natural and artificial. Getting at least 30 minutes of natural daylight during the daytime is vital for setting your bodily rhythm. So, make sure you let light into your day so you can sleep better and dream bigger at night.

- Watch your stress levels during the day, as stress is the enemy of not just your physical and mental health, but your dream health too. Find ways to relax. An overcrowded life won't just chase your waking calm away, but those dream memories too.

- Avoid screen time an hour before sleeping, as computers, TVs and mobiles overstimulate your brain and prevent the release of sleep-inducing hormones.

- It is important you calm down and avoid any physical and mental stress at least an hour before bed. Journalling, chatting to loved ones, indulging in a warm bath, savouring herbal tea or anything else that relaxes you is ideal.

- Try a spot of video-gaming. Around 30 minutes a day can work a treat for your memory and brain health and for igniting dream recall, because in a video-game you are immersing yourself in an different reality, practising for the dream state. Just be sure to game in moderation and avoid doing it two hours before bedtime.

⊕ If gaming isn't your thing, 30 minutes of reading fiction before bedtime will also spark your dreaming mind. Einstein, who valued imagination more than knowledge, once said, 'If you want your children to be intelligent, let them read fairy stories.' Reading is dreaming with eyes wide open.

⊕ Do some backwards thinking. In the dream state there is no concept of time, so a simple warm-up exercise you can do at any time during the day is to remember the events of your last 24 hours backwards. This will send a clear signal to your dreaming mind that you are willing to ditch logic and addiction to linear time and enter into a dialogue with it. *Warning*: Thinking backwards isn't as easy as it sounds. You may only manage it in 10-second bursts at first, as your conscious mind will constantly step in to impose linear order.

⊕ Cultivate a curious mindset. Embrace new perspectives. Learn a new language. Try a different route to work, a new restaurant, or a new recipe. Sit in a different chair. Shake up your daily routine. Do one thing that surprises you each day. Give your dreaming mind stand-out moments in your day so it has plenty of food to nourish it at night. Your dreams are very closely linked to how you process emotion and store memories. If your waking life is a curious, open-minded one and you are willing to learn new things, consider different perspectives and get comfortable outside your comfort zone, this will dramatically increase your chances of vivid dream recall.

The Stuff of your Dreams

Find your dream balance

Your dream life and waking life are interconnected. You are going to dream about your waking life and, after reading this book, your waking life is going to be infused with the vision of your dreams.

Sometimes poor dream recall is a sign that you need to look at your waking life first and find greater balance between your intuition and creativity and your logic and reason. Perhaps your life has got too busy, too clock-driven or too dependent on data or validations from other people and things. In short, your worth is coming from the outside in, rather than from the inside out. Your dreaming mind feels abandoned.

Daily meditation is one way to restore that balance between intuition and logic. If the 'm' word alarms you, don't let it. As you'll see in the dream-inducing meditation on page 69, you don't have to contort yourself in uncomfortable positions for hours to meditate, all you need to do is take some time to be fully present. Focusing on your breath for a few minutes is a simple way to do this. If busy thoughts come in, just notice them and don't interact with them. And of course, every time you recall a dream and let it play out behind your eyes without judging or interacting with it in any way, you are entering an observant semi-meditative state. You are witnessing your mindset.

Alternatively, you can listen to relaxing music before you go to sleep. This is such a great way to find inner calm, because when you listen to music your logical mind is listening to the notes, seeking a pattern, leaving your unconscious mind free to do what it does best – daydream. Your conscious and unconscious selves are walking side by side, doing what they do best, and not disagreeing or minimizing each other. Result: inner calm.

The inability to recall dreams is the mightiest roadblock to dream work and it may take a few weeks to clear. But above all, don't try to force those dream memories to come. They will come when they feel you are ready.

NONSENSE

Following poor dream recall, the next biggest dream-work roadblock is struggling to understand your dreams.

If you can recall your dreams but have given up trying to make sense of them, the following lessons will help you become your own dream oracle. But as you work through them, please bear in mind that sometimes you may still get a dream that defies all your attempts at decoding it, however much you brainstorm it. This is nothing to worry about and everything to get overjoyed about. The infinite mystery of dreams is their beauty. As you'll find, as soon as you try to define them by a set of rules, they shapeshift into something else. I often compare them to the ocean and to outer space. You can learn to sail across the ocean, but you can never completely control it. It is possible to journey into space, too, but there is so much about it we can't understand or even reach yet.

So, on the rare occasions when you recall a dream which, despite your best efforts, is beyond your understanding, simply thank your dreaming mind for reminding you of the infinite creative potential within you. Ask for more clarity next time.

And bear in mind that sometimes your dreaming mind may just want to take you on a wild nocturnal adventure for the sheer fun of it – to remind you to lighten up and take yourself a little less seriously.

NO TIME

Another roadblock is not having enough time in the morning to write down your dreams.

A voice recorder you can speak into is a great way to get round this, but if you prefer pen and paper, write down the first dream that comes into your mind. If that means letting the other dreams go, so be it. This one has surfaced first for a reason.

A couple of minutes should be all you need. Indeed, it is preferable, as less can often be more when it comes to decoding your dreams later in the day. If you haven't got a few minutes first thing, you may want to reassess what matters to you and why you aren't prioritizing the wealth of bespoke creativity within you.

When recording your dreams, stick to time-saving key words rather than lengthy descriptions.

You might also want to try drawing your dreams, and if you truly feel stuck, sometimes an AI image-maker app where you input your dreams to see what image it creates can ignite connections or perspectives you might not have considered before.

Note: You may find that as you work through this book, you start to experience dream overcrowding. This is a clear sign your dreaming mind is excited about connecting with you and has a lot it wants to share with you. Don't tell it to send you fewer dreams, just focus on the two or three dreams that shout the loudest.

UNSETTLING DREAMS

Last, but by no means least, you may be reluctant to linger with your dreams on waking because the content feels unsettling or disturbing. Join the dream club. The majority of dreams are anxiety-based, because the primary function of dreaming is problem-solving and problems are the engine that drive our lives forward. If your dreams feel toxic or verge into nightmare territory, it is doubly important for you to recall them and work out what they want you to know. Your dreaming mind is pointing to areas of pain in your waking life to teach you something you need to learn so you can move beyond it.

Your dreams are a symbolic reflection of your own mindset, and should what you see or experience in them make you feel anxious, the solution is to make changes in your waking mindset so your dreams start reflecting inner empowerment back to you. The more empowering your dreams are, the more rewarding your waking life will be.

Of course, as you should be sensing by now, your dreams love to tear up any rule-book, so even if you feel you have a deeply satisfying waking life, on occasion an unsettling dream scenario may still startle you on waking, for the simple reason it's good for your personal growth.

Dreams train you to expect the unexpected. You don't learn, move and grow in what is safe and predictable. So, your dreaming mind wants to keep you constantly challenged. The wind needs to be against the plane when it takes off, not with it. Having said that, if you are reflective in your waking life and making strides in your personal growth, chances are your dreams will reflect that fulfilment back to you in joyful spades.

Hopelessly devoted to you

Although your night vision has many superpowers – it can problem-solve, release creative blocks, glimpse potential futures, and so on – perhaps its greatest power is its ability to help you understand yourself better. Hopelessly devoted to your well-being, your dreams truly are personal growth wishes your heart makes on your behalf every night.

If someone tells me they don't understand the meaning of their dreams, in my opinion what they are saying is that at a deep unconscious level they don't understand themselves. And if they say they can't be bothered to recall their dreams, or don't see the point, it suggests lack of interest in their own personal growth. If people say these kinds of things to me, these days I don't try to convince them of their own dream power. Instead, I simply ask them to harvest 20 or more of their dreams and then check back in with me at a later date. In almost every case, when they check back in and we discuss the potential meanings of their dreams, a light bulb goes on.

During the day, most of us rarely stop to process and make sense of our emotional and mental reactions to external events. Every dream recalled is a precious opportunity for greater self-awareness. There is hidden treasure to be discovered in every single surreal story, scene, image, colour, sound, feeling and object. All you need to do is recall and record your dreams and then reflect on what they have to teach you.

From now on, start thinking of your dreaming mind as your best friend who is also your mentor and teacher. Every dream takes you right back to your personal growth night school, offering you something valuable to help you evolve. And the absolute must-have night-school text book is your dream journal.

RECORDING YOUR DREAMS

The first rule of dream work is to record your dreams. The second rule is to record your dreams.

Your dream journal is the book of your soul, a sacred artefact.

Keeping a dream journal is non-negotiable when it comes to interpreting what your night vision wants you to know. You *have* to document your dreams, because, as explained previously, if you don't, they will slip away from your memory forever, taking all their precious personal illumination and stunning creativity with them.

If you have never kept a dream journal before or haven't made it a morning ritual yet, before reading any more of this book, please commit to keeping one immediately. Don't panic if that feels like another thing to do. It just takes two minutes every morning, is a gift for your personal growth and can be tremendously rewarding.

And if you have already been keeping a dream journal, bravo! Please keep that safe, but may I politely ask you to draw a line under it and restart your dream documenting afresh.

Take 20

Tonight, before you go to bed, simply put a blank sheet of paper and a pen beside your bed, along with a night light or torch to use if it is too dark to write anything down when you wake up. Don't immediately go for a dream notebook, as there is something very enticing about a single blank page with a pen close by. It is asking you to write, and that's what you need to start getting into the habit of doing. Although 'habit' isn't quite the right word, as that implies doing something mindlessly, without conscious thought. So, let's replace 'habit' with 'ritual'.

Rituals are things you choose to do repeatedly with sacred intention and awareness. Aristotle is believed to have stated, 'You are what you repeatedly do,' and if you repeatedly write down your dreams on waking, you are a dream oracle.

On waking, when dream memories surface, write down the date and any symbols or feelings that come to mind.

To help you record your dreams in the optimum way, turn to page 261, where there is a template for recording the first 20, when the emphasis is on simply recalling them and writing them down. Give that template a try for a day or so and then, if you feel it is wanting, make personal adjustments.

Once you have recorded your dream memories, put your piece of paper away in a file, drawer or somewhere safe and go about your day. The morning isn't the time to decode your dreams.

I'm actually going to suggest that you don't start interpreting your dreams at all until you have harvested at least 20. This means placing a blank piece of paper and a pen at your bedside every night for at least the next 20 nights. If you wake up one morning with no dream recall, simply write that down anyway. This is important, because it will reinforce the ritual of dream journalling. Remember, you are what you repeatedly do.

The reason I am asking you to collect 20 dreams before you even start the work of decoding them is that dreams work as a series, often commenting on each other, and you need to get that message. Too many of us focus on one dream and forget that the following night there will be the next thrilling instalment of your edge-of-the-seat personal growth adventures. You need to tune in every night for all the plot twists and revelations.

It is tempting to start decoding your dreams immediately, and there is nothing to stop you doing so. But I would advise patience, as it takes time for seeds to grow in the darkness.

Also, it is very important that you start relishing the feeling of waking up with dreams on your mind and simply enjoy the process of writing them down, without expectation. Focusing too much on analysis or forcing interpretations in the early days of keeping a dream journal can kill your enthusiasm and drive your beautiful dreams away. You first need to prove to yourself that you are a dreaming being, and the optimum way to do that is to record at least 20 of your dreams.

DREAM READING

I hope you will often revisit these 20 dreams, recorded at a time when you recommitted yourself to dream work. The dream seeds you plant now will set things in motion.

Reading your dreams in hindsight can be a revelation, but sadly it is the crucial thing many people forget to do. This is a pity, because the best dream book is always the one you write yourself. Oscar Wilde once said he always needed something sensational to read on a train, so he brought his own diary. I'm going to better that and say your dream cure journal is going to be your sensational must-read from now on.

Dream reading

On the afternoon or early evening after you have recalled and recorded your twentieth dream, find somewhere quiet where you won't be disturbed, gather your 20 dreams together, in the order that you dreamed them, and read your sensational story so far. Please don't try to make sense of these dreams. Simply celebrate them as evidence that you are alive from the inside out with the vision, creativity and guidance of your dreams.

You might want to lay the 20 pieces of paper out on the floor like a spreadsheet or a design plan. Seeing them all laid out before you in this way is quite something. You may even feel inspired to give your inside-out narrative a title.

Reading your dreams as a 20-part series will underline to you that your dreams are an ongoing narrative. Too many people get obsessed with one particularly vivid dream, forgetting that the following night another dream will comment on it and add further insight. Remember, you need to approach your dreams in the same way as you would if you invested your time in watching a long-running TV series, where each episode deepened the plot and you learned more about the characters and the direction of the narrative. With your dreams, you need to tune in night after night to find out what happens next in the unmissable story of you and your personal growth. Trust me, it's going to be the greatest show on Earth!

Writing the book of your soul

If you used loose sheets of paper for your first 20 dream recalls, store them somewhere safe so you can return to them at any time, but you don't have to include them in your journal going forward. This reminds you that your dreaming mind is not limited, but a bottomless pit of never-ending creativity. There are always bigger and better dreams to come.

Your dream journal

If you haven't already done so, now is the time to invest in a dream journal. If you struggle to read your own writing, as I often do these days, you might want to consider a voice recorder. Should you decide to write down your dreams, try to make sure your journal is hardback, to reflect the gravitas of your dreams.

Before you go to bed, bless that journal simply by placing your hands on it and put it on your bedside table or somewhere you can immediately see and reach on waking.

Choose a pen that is smooth and flowing to write with and place it beside your journal.

Morning

Then every morning, after following the dream-recall tips on page 42, dedicate two side-by-side blank pages of your journal to one day. Divide those two pages into four quarters: two on the left-hand side and two on the right-hand side. To help you set this in motion, on page 262 you will find a template to follow.

Write the date on the top part of the left-hand page and underneath document your dreams according to the guidelines given in the template. Resist the temptation to go into lengthy descriptions. A couple of minutes is all this should take. Stick to key words and feelings and any personal associations that immediately come to mind. Writing down your dreams in the present rather than the past tense can help you keep the dream alive and remind you that your dreams are always current. They are commenting on what is happening in your life right now.

You may also want to draw rather than write down some of the images from your dreams.

Resist the temptation to try to turn your dreams into a linear or logical story with a beginning, middle and end, or to make sense of them. First thing in the morning your attitude should simply be one of open-minded acceptance of your dreams and, most important of all, gratitude for the inner healing they bring. Trust that when the time is right you will understand what they have to say.

After you have written down the key words and feelings of your dream, see if any personal associations come to mind and record them in the bottom half of the left-hand page. Don't spend too long on this; simply go with your first impressions, however nonsensical and random, and if there are none, that is fine too.

If you notice recurring themes or symbols in your dreams, take note, as they are recurring for a reason. They are drawing your attention to something painful or conflicting in your waking life because you still need to learn the lesson that these experiences teach. When you do understand and learn, those dreams will cease.

Waking with little or no recollection of your dreams is no reason not to write in your dream journal. It can help to write the words 'I feel' and then write down how you feel, because that feeling will have been inspired by a dream.

You can also reread a previous dream, or return to your original 20 dreams, and reflect on what associations those dreams went on to inspire. Doing this can prompt the dream-recall part of your brain.

You could also write something along the lines of:

My dream memories aren't clear at the moment, but I look forward to my next dream recall.

The Stuff of your Dreams

Whatever you decide to do, make sure you write something, anything, in your dream journal every morning.

Daytime

Then go about your day as normal.

Should any more dream memories or associations surface, document them. And every time you document any feeling, image, or story from your dreaming mind, thank your unconscious for the insight and associations that this is going to ignite within you.

Evening

Later in the day, ideally in the evening before you go to bed, set aside around five to ten minutes for your dream work.

Return to your dream journal or file. If you have had any other impressions filtering through in the day, add them in on the left-hand side of the page.

Then, on the top half of the right-hand side of the page, write down – again using key words – significant things that have happened to you during the day. If it has been a quiet day, be sure to write that down too.

This documenting of the events in your day on the right-hand part of the page is very important for your dream work, as it will give you a sense of how your dreams are foreshadowing or commenting on your waking life.

When you have written down the key events of your day on the top right-hand side of the page, focus on the images, feelings and symbols from your previous night's dream that jump out at you or the ones you feel instinctively drawn to. I would suggest keeping these symbols down to no more than three. These three symbols will jump out at you for a reason, and that is to tell you something about yourself that you need to know for your personal growth.

Seeing your dream life and your waking life presented side by side for the first time is a profound experience. You begin to see clearly how there is a symbolic poetic voiceover or nocturnal narrative endlessly commenting on and complementing your waking life. One fun technique I encourage is to think what that dream voiceover would sound like. You can assign it any voice you like – that of a celebrity or a fictional character, an animal sound or your own voice.

The bottom half of the right-hand page is reserved for your own dream decoding. You may want to write down a question about the dominant symbols you have noticed and record any answers or impressions that come to you. You can also write down any personal associations or connections that come to you.

Later on

When you have documented your dream life and waking life side by side for several days, you can look back to the events of the day (or days) before to see how your dreams are always trying to help you problem-solve and make sense of things. You may also see how they foreshadow your future. And if elements of your dream have played out in your waking life, be sure to make a note of it.

You can't get a sense of your dreaming mind watching over you with your best interests at heart until you actually see in hindsight your waking and dream life placed side by side in your dream journal.

As for decoding your dreams, read on, as the next lesson is devoted to the optimum way to go about brainstorming the personal meaning of your dreams.

For now, just ensure you are writing something (even something very brief) in your journal every morning and evening. You're gathering data.

BECOMING A DREAM SCIENTIST

Your dream journal is your data, your scientific proof that your dreams matter. As long as you write down your dreams and parallel them with your waking life, you can return to them at any point to do some decoding. You don't have to do this right away. Sometimes rereading a dream you had weeks or months or even years ago is a Eureka moment, triggering an insight that is profoundly healing. Indeed, decoding your dreams with the benefit of hindsight is something I recommend highly.

And while on the theme of hindsight, do keep on looking back at your past dreams. Chances are you'll notice themes that keep repeating, and they will keep repeating until you have learned what they are trying to teach you.

I've kept a dream journal from childhood. I have a vast library of dream journals now, as you can imagine, and it's the most fascinating reading that I do. If you are familiar with the concept of the Akashic records, it does feel as if I'm not just reading the book of my life, but of my soul. That's why I urge you, if you want to write down your dreams rather than type them in a document or speak them into a voice recorder, to make sure your dream journals have strong or attractive covers, so they have the feel of a wonderful library.

If I notice themes from my childhood dreams that I am still dreaming about all these decades later, I double down on trying to decode their personal meaning and aim to apply what I discover to my waking life. And when those themes become less frequent in my current dreams, I know that I am finally learning what those dreams wanted me to know from childhood onwards. For some reason I haven't got the message until now, but at last I've removed a roadblock to my personal growth. It's an incredibly liberating feeling.

If you haven't kept a dream journal from childhood, you don't need to go back to dreams you had decades ago to get this feeling. Simply recognizing a repeating dream theme from a week or so before and uncovering what that theme is trying to teach you can have the same empowering impact on your waking life.

I hope that by now you understand how vital keeping a dream journal is for your dream work. It's a powerful signal to your dreaming mind that you are committed to gathering proof as a citizen oneirologist that your dreams matter. Trust me, your dreaming mind will take note of your commitment to it – it notices everything you think, feel and do during the day – and from the moment you start documenting your night visions, it won't fail to reward you with endless illuminations when the time is right.

Now that you are primed for dream recall, understand the importance of writing in your dream journal every day and are getting to grips with the optimum way to write down your dreams, there are just a few more preliminaries to consider before you plunge into the wild and wonderful world of dream decoding.

SEASONAL CONSIDERATIONS

Let's first consider seasonal transitions and their impact on your dream life. During the summer your body can overheat, which increases the likelihood of more anxious-themed dreams and clearer dream recall. During heatwaves, the heat can also cause lighter sleep, meaning you are more likely to wake up during REM with vivid dream recall.

Memorable and vivid dreams can also occur during seasonal transitions and whenever your body clock is unsettled by clocks going backwards or forwards or by overseas travel. One of the most common dream themes when the season changes is dreaming of being lost – a symbol of uncertainty.

The day of the week may also be influential, as studies show that people are more likely to recall their dreams on Friday or over the weekend, the reason being that you may have a more leisurely morning on those days if you follow a traditional working week, and lingering in bed a while longer on waking may encourage dream recall.

DREAM POSITIONING

Something else that can impact your dream life is the position you sleep in. Are you a front, back or side sleeper? Each position comes with its own pros and cons that you might want to consider next time you tumble into bed.

There is no overall consensus about which sleeping position is optimum for dream recall, but the limited studies that have been done suggest it's sleeping on your side. Sleeping on your back may be associated with an increased risk of nightmares, and this could be connected to the impact of back sleeping on breathing. Issues with breathing can cause poor-quality sleep, and whenever there is poor-quality sleep, the chances of anxiety-themed dreaming increases.

Stomach sleeping isn't bad news – indeed, some studies have shown stomach sleepers have more sensual dreams – but if I had to choose a position most likely to induce dream recall and those dreams being cathartic and healing, it would be side sleeping, with the right side just edging it over the left, as left-sided sleeping may put stress on the heart, although bear in mind that if you suffer from reflux, right-side sleeping may not be optimum. You might want to write down the sleeping position you wake up in when you have dream recall to see if that plays a part in boosting recall. But remember that when it comes to dream work, sufficient quality sleep is way more important than the position you prefer.

FOOD AND DRINK

Contrary to what you may have been led to believe, eating cheese before you go to sleep isn't going to give you nightmares, but eating anything, whether it is cheese rich or not, right before you go to sleep is going to influence your dream life. Nocturnal meals require your body to focus on digestion rather than winding down physically for a good night's sleep. After a large meal, your sleep may be lighter and you may find that you wake up several times during the night with anxiety-themed dream memories. So, eating late at night will also lead to fatigue on waking. Not to mention that it's far better to just have one or two dream images on waking than countless distressing ones.

Alcohol is another sleep-disruptor, and whenever sleep is poor, your body dips in and out of the important sleep stages and dream quality is compromised. You won't reach the deep unconscious state that nourishes your dreaming mind; instead your conscious waking mind may remain too dominant, resulting in hallucinations.

Ideally, you should avoid eating supper any later than two hours before bedtime. A light snack or milky drink or herbal tea before bedtime can be comforting, but ensure it is light. And most important of all, avoid alcohol, as it is toxic for your bloodstream, your mind and your chances of quality sleep.

THIEF OF DREAMS

Also avoid using your mobile or laptop or watching TV for at least an hour before bedtime, as the light from the screens will mess with your sleep schedule. If you have got into the habit of watching TV in the evening until you feel sleepy, this may be your biggest challenge, but to get the most out of your dream work you have to let go of those screens.

Instead of watching TV immediately before you go to bed, study your dream journal, take a bath, spend time with loved ones or pets, or best of all read this book, or any book, although fiction would be ideal, instead. If you have a TV in your bedroom, consider moving it somewhere else.

The same goes for your mobile phone. Stop using it and place it on silent at least an hour before bedtime. At night, put it in a drawer, or better still, charge it in a different room. And avoid the routine of checking your phone first thing when you wake up. Give yourself at least half an hour before you grab your attention-seeking phone, with all the demands and messages coming from others and not from you.

You may want to write in your journal the time you stop using screens before you go to sleep to see how it impacts your dream life.

CRYSTALS AND CATCHERS

In addition to placing your dream-life journal on your bedside table every night, you may also want to consider placing a dream-enhancing crystal or dream-catcher somewhere in your bedroom.

Amethyst is believed to boost dream recall and promote a good night's sleep, due to its alleged calming effect on the mind, and the calmer and more relaxed you are on waking, the better your dream recall will be.

Rose quartz may help you have sweet dreams. It is a crystal associated with unconditional love. You might want to hold it in your hand before you go to sleep and ask your dreaming mind to send you positive dreams.

A dream-catcher may help put you in a calm and optimistic frame of mind before you go to sleep. Dream-catchers are typically nets decorated with feathers and beads that are believed to have the spiritual power to catch bad dreams and only let good ones through. These beautiful protective items were once an integral part of Native American culture, and especially popular among the Dakota and Cree.

Crystals and dream-catchers are eye-catching and add a certain mystic ambience to a bedroom, but they are by no means essential. You may have noticed the word 'belief' used rather frequently when discussing their alleged powers. Although there are plenty of anecdotal reports that testify to this power, the real power lies in your belief. Mindset is key. If you believe a certain crystal or dream-catcher is going to protect you and bring you healing dreams, it might do just that.

SCENT OF A DREAM

Studies show that external stimuli, such as scents, can have an impact on your dream life. If you feel stressed or anxious, your chances of disrupted sleep and nightmares skyrocket. So, using essential oils, like lavender, camomile, rosemary, peppermint and bergamot, that are believed to have calming properties can help you have a better night's sleep and may even reduce the chances of nightmares.

One dream recall-inducing essential oil you might want to experiment with by adding a few drops on your pillow before you go to sleep or by adding to a diffuser is mugwort. The Chumash Native Americans named this plant 'dream sage'.

Smells are processed by your brain's limbic system, which also deals with your memory and your emotions, and the thing with scent is that it is a very personal experience. So you need to test the power of scent out for yourself to monitor its impact on your dream life.

TALK TO YOURSELF

Before you go to sleep each night, give yourself a little talking-to. Tell your dreaming mind gently but assertively that you are looking forward to the dreams that will come and to recalling them in the morning.

Salvador Dalí once described his artwork as photographs of his dreams. He would wake from a sleep or a nap with images on his mind and would instantly write them down because he knew that if he didn't document them straight away, they would vanish and take their magical creativity with them.

So, let this be another reminder to always have your dream journal close by when you fall asleep, so you can immediately 'photograph' in some way your dreams on waking, even if that waking is in the middle of the night. You simply won't remember if you put it off or do something else, such as drinking a glass of water or brushing your teeth.

MEDITATION

Anything that reduces your stress levels in waking life is not only good news for your physical, emotional and mental health, but also for your sleep and dream health.

Meditation isn't for everyone, but it has been shown to be a mighty stress-buster. You might want to consider incorporating it into your day or your evening routine, because there is a valid connection between daily meditation and a vivid dream life. Interestingly, people who say they don't recall their dreams typically do after a couple of weeks of daily meditation. It seems that meditation wakes up the part of the brain associated with intuition, imagination and creativity – and therefore dream recall.

Meditation truly isn't complicated and it is a shame so many courses make it appear so. It is actually very simple. It is simply setting aside a few minutes a day in a place where you can be safely alone and undisturbed. Then get comfortable, close your eyes and start focusing your thoughts on your breath. Breathe in calm and breathe out anxiety. If thoughts interrupt, notice them but don't interact with them. Indeed, meditation isn't the absence of thought that many people believe it to be, it is detaching from thoughts and observing them. You don't judge or fear whatever your mind wants to tell you. You just notice.

You could compare meditation to sitting beside a stream and watching it flow by. Your thoughts and your emotions are the stream, but you are separate from them and able to observe them without judgement.

In this way, a spot of daily meditation helps you separate your thoughts from your body and become more observant of yourself and your reality when you are awake. And the more aware you are during the day, the more vivid your dreams will be at night.

You just need to find a meditation technique that works for you. You may be one of those people who find that reading a good book, listening to beautiful music, stroking a beloved pet, singing or tidying up is an effective meditation alternative. However, if you want to give meditation a go, just commit to three to five minutes of 'quiet time' each day, ideally before you go to sleep.

I'm using the words 'quiet time' here rather than 'mindfulness' and 'meditation', as they can have time-consuming associations and you may be one of those people who don't like to be told to slow down. However, if you want to have amazing dream recall, setting aside a few minutes of quiet time, ideally before you go to bed, to connect to the invisible intuitive, creative part of yourself that never sleeps and is wide awake in your dreams is a real dream-recall booster.

Five minutes of quiet time

Set a timer for five minutes.

Find somewhere to sit quietly and comfortably with your back straight and your hands relaxed in your lap.

Half-close your eyes and look downwards.

Tell yourself to be still and breathe slowly from your stomach rather than your chest.

Be sure to breathe in slowly through your nose, and then, when your lungs are full, to exhale slowly and completely through your mouth. Notice how it feels when air enters your nostrils and sails down your throat into your lungs. Concentrate on the sensations when you exhale and notice how every inhale and every exhale is different. No two breaths are the same.

Focus gently on breathing in and out, and as you do so, notice how many thoughts and feelings start screaming for your attention.

The Stuff of your Dreams

Don't ignore those thoughts or interact with them in any way; just let them pass through you.

When the timer goes off, fully close your eyes and, still looking downwards, imagine you are looking deep into your own heart and soul.

If you see anything, make a mental note of it, but if you see nothing, that is absolutely fine.

Gently return to looking straight ahead and then open your eyes and congratulate yourself on successfully completing five minutes of quiet time.

You may notice that it was refreshing to take time out from your attention-grabbing thoughts. This is because you have been reminded that your thoughts and feelings do not define or own you, just as your body does not define you either. You have connected to who you really are, the invisible part of yourself you are going to meet in your dreams.

If you find this exercise calming and helpful for boosting dream recall, you can repeat it twice a day, but don't fall into the trap of thinking that the longer you meditate, the more progress you will make. Quality, not quantity, is key when it comes to meditation, and sleep and dream work.

MINDFULNESS

You may want to complement your daily dream-inducing meditation with a mindfulness exercise. Mindfulness isn't quite the same as meditation, but it can be equally healing and beneficial for both your waking and dreaming life. The difference is that in meditation you pause to calm and clear your mind by observing your thoughts, but in mindfulness you carry on with your routine but become fully present and aware of your external surroundings as well as your inner world of thoughts and feelings.

As with meditation, mindfulness is very simple and you really don't need to go on courses and retreats to learn it. Just start doing it the next time you take a walk.

Walking mindfully

Dedicate five minutes of your walking time to focusing on nothing but the steps you are taking and the surroundings you are walking through.

Focus on the feeling of your feet as they hit the ground, your legs as they move, your arms as they swing, your head as it directs the whole procedure.

And when those pesky thoughts intervene (trust me, they will), just notice them and let them walk on by.

Then expand your awareness to noticing your surroundings. Use all your senses. Take in all those tiny details you would normally miss. Look at the world around you like a detective in search of hidden clues.

Research has shown that daily meditation can influence the shape of your brain, strengthening key areas of the cortex associated with attention, concentration, memory and reflection. And whatever reshapes your brain will show up in your dreams.

THE BEGINNING OF ALL HEALING

Writing down your dreams – or thinking about the possibilities of your dreams, if recall is poor – is the perfect start to each new day. It sets a sacred tone and is an assertive statement to yourself and the universe of your commitment to your personal growth and healing.

Indeed, it is the ultimate act of self-respect and self-care. You are paying attention to what your unconscious wants you to know. You are showing yourself first thing that your personal growth and healing are your absolute priority. You are working on understanding and healing yourself from the inside out. You are conscious that the greatest relationship of all – and the one that sets the tone for all your other relationships and everything you attract into your life – is the relationship you have with yourself and your dreams. Not working on that loving relationship with yourself is the biggest cause of all unhappiness and feelings of emptiness in the world.

It wouldn't be an understatement to say that dream work, with the self-awareness it brings and the self-care and inner magic it inspires, is the real secret to lasting happiness.

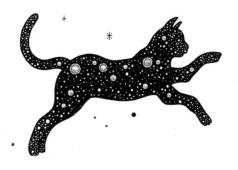

HOW TO INTERPRET YOUR DREAMS

Night light: Understanding the meaning of your dreams is understanding your unconscious beliefs about yourself and whether those unconscious beliefs are increasing or decreasing your chances of happiness.

If you visit a country where people speak a different language, the best way to truly understand and communicate with them is to learn it. That's how you need to think about dreaming. The world of your dreams is a different state of consciousness and the language there is completely different from your waking one.

This lesson is designed to help you learn the language of dreams as quickly as possible.

BEYOND THE OBVIOUS

Don't be daunted. Learning dream language isn't quite as time-consuming and arduous as learning a foreign language. This is because it is a language that your ancestors spoke fluently, and it's likely that you did too when you were a child, but you may have lost your grasp of it as you got older. It is the instinctive language of your heart, which is the language of emotions expressed in symbols.

In ancient times we had an intuitive grasp of this deep language and the way it helped us look beneath the surface for deeper meaning. However, over time, with the fast pace of industry and online life overriding our connection with nature, electricity unnaturally extending our waking hours and the advance of science diminishing the role of intuition in our lives, it is a language many have forgotten how to speak. But your dreams haven't forgotten, and neither have many poets, artists, musicians and visionaries.

Cast your memory back to your schooldays. At some point it's likely that your teacher gave you a poem to interpret. Your task was to spot the associated or deeper meanings behind the literal words, revealed through the poet's use of symbolism and figurative language. And you would have found, as all students of poetry do, that symbols not only have common or universal meanings, but they also carry an infinite number of personal associations.

So, here is a shift which will immediately help you understand your dreams better. From now on, start thinking of them in the same way you would interpret a poem or a work of art. Words often have limits. Symbols don't. We've all heard the saying 'a picture paints a thousand words' – well the visions in your dreams paint thousands too.

You may not think of yourself as a poet or artist, but in your dreams you are the greatest night poet and artist you know.

STOP AND STARE

If you haven't watched the movie *Inception* yet, it's a must-watch. It's directed by a visionary filmmaker and self-confessed lucid dreamer, Christopher Nolan. It doesn't get everything right about dream power, but it gets a whole lot right, has a thrilling storyline and is a cinematic treat. You really feel as if you are entering the world of the dream. I am referencing this movie as it contains an iconic scene where everyone in the dream stops and stares at the dreamer. This showcases beautifully how your dream symbolism talks to you.

Almost everything in your dream – the people, the location, the story, the objects, the colours, the sensations, the sounds, and so on – symbolizes an aspect of your own mindset. It really is all about you. It's like a hall of mirrors, only you create the hall, the mirrors and what they reflect back at you. And once you understand that your dreams and everything that goes on in them are almost always about *you*, your dream interpretation will take a giant leap forward.

When you want to interpret a dream, the first place you may look may be the interpretations given online or in book form. These can be helpful, as they ignite symbolic thinking. However, you are always the best person to understand the meaning of the symbols in your dreams, whatever anyone else says. For example, if you adore cats and dream of one, it would be a symbol of loving companionship, as well as mystery and independence. However, if you dislike cats or are allergic to them, the appearance of one in a dream will have the opposite interpretation.

So, always go for your gut instinct or personal emotional association with a dream symbol first. Write down in your dream journal the very first thing that comes into your mind when you reflect on it, however bizarre or unrelated that association may seem. If nothing at all comes to mind, focus on the feeling you associate with that symbol and write that down.

RETRACE YOUR STEPS

Just before I share with you the specifics of personal dream decoding, let's retrace our steps a little, because the following reminders need to be firmly in place first:

1. Whenever you go to sleep or take a nap, have your dream journal – whether that is a notebook, file or voice recorder – within reach, ready for when you wake up. You may also want to have a pen with a light at the ready if it will be dark when you wake up. However you decide to record your dreams, make sure you have plenty of space to do it in.

Empty space waiting to be filled is an open invitation your dreaming mind is unlikely to ignore.

2. As you fall asleep, welcome in your dreams with your thoughts. You might want to clench your entire body and then relax it, particularly your facial muscles, as many of us frown when we are awake without even realizing it. Relaxation is optimum for drifting off to sleep, which is a highly suggestible state, so make the most of it by telling yourself you are going to recall your dreams on waking.

3. If you wake up in the middle of the night with a dream on your mind, write down some key words from it immediately. Don't tell yourself you'll remember it in the morning, because you won't.

4. On waking, ideally without an alarm clock, don't immediately jump out of bed. Stay still for a minute or two and let those dream memories surface. Then write them down before starting your day.

5. No dream is too trivial or nonsensical to write down. There is always some deep insight hiding there. Having said that, if you experience dream overcrowding and haven't got time to write pages of dream notes each day on waking, focus on what commands your attention the most. Discipline yourself to recording the three strongest memories.

6. Be sure to write the date of the dream, as this may prove to be very significant in hindsight.

How to Interpret your Dreams

7. If you wake up knowing you had a dream but it just isn't surfacing in your memory, let it go. Trying to trap a butterfly in your hand can kill it. If the message that dream has for you is important, it will resurface the following night or the night after that.

8. As you write down your dreams, feel deep gratitude for every symbol and record the immediate associations each symbol has for you. Don't be tempted to explain away dream symbols because you have been reading a book or watching a movie or the news and symbols from that book, movie, etc., appeared in your dream. Your dreaming mind is super clever, and of all the countless symbols you encountered that day, it chose those specific ones for a reason. Your job is to become your own dream detective and find out why.

9. Always try to relate your dream theme to your current waking life.

DECODING YOUR NEXT DREAM

The next time you wake up with dream memories on your mind, write them down and feel ready to begin decoding them in earnest, wait. Please wait until the evening, ideally just before you go to bed. This the perfect time to think about the meaning of your dreams, because the bustle of the day is over, you are likely to be feeling relaxed and you'll now have the opportunity to connect the day's events with the previous night's dream. Last, but by no means least, thinking about dreams before you fall asleep, when your mind is super-suggestible, is a great way to boost recall the next morning. Fall asleep and wake up with dreams on your mind!

The dream cure decoding template below will give your dream-decoding work a structure. As you decode, be sure to reference the prompts below. Keep referring to them until the decoding work you do every evening in your dream journal becomes second nature.

DECODING PROMPTS

1. In the overwhelming majority of cases, dreams are symbolic, but there's no harm ruling out a literal interpretation.

2. Consider the dream as a symbolic representation of your current mindset. Your dreams comment on your current waking reality, though sometimes they may use symbols and themes from your past or childhood to do so. But even when dreams take you back in time, they will have been created by and be commenting on something that is *currently* weighing on your mind. Consider your identity in the dream and whether you are an observer (which suggests the need to be more objective and see the bigger picture) or an active participant.

3. Less is more. Minimize your word count. Focus on key words. Choose one to three key symbols or themes and focus your interpretation on those initially. Go for those that feel dominant or you recalled most clearly on waking or feel most drawn to. They are right at the top of your dream

inbox for a reason. As you select these keywords/themes, be guided by those that ignite the strongest emotion and which resonate most with your current waking reality. If nothing resonates, notice in coming days moments when scenes, objects or emotions from your dream feature in your waking life. Your dreams often have precognitive elements.

4. Consider your personal associations with a specific dream theme or symbol *before* investigating the common, universal or abstract ones. If you don't have any personal associations and decide to search online or in a book, this can be a helpful way to kick-start symbolic thinking. But do take universal interpretations as a possible meaning, not the definitive one.

5. Your dreams don't want to tell you what you already know about yourself, and if you come to this conclusion, you need to dig deeper. Your dreams *are* all about you, but they aren't your echo chamber. Their purpose is to offer new perspectives and tell you something about yourself that you don't know. Your dreams love to surprise you.

6. Go through all the possible interpretations and notice the one that feels the most elevating or expansive, gives you goose bumps or a moment of clarity, or inspires you to take positive action in your waking life. That will be the correct interpretation. If the interpretation you settle on drains or diminishes you in any way, it is not the correct one. Like your best friend, your dreams only want to raise you up.

7. When you have considered as many interpretations as you can and settled on one that speaks to you, write that down in your dream journal in one or two sentences. *Be sure to always make your personal dream decoding as positive and as empowering as possible.* The chapters that follow will show you that every dream symbol, however terrifying, shocking or dismal, carries the potential for a positive interpretation. Your role as your own dream detective is to zone in on that positive interpretation time and time and time again. Positivity is your new dream interpretation mantra. View every fresh insight from your deep that surfaces into your waking awareness with gratitude for how it can help you learn, heal and evolve.

8. Then write down what practical empowering thing(s) you intend to do about it in your waking life. The purpose of your dreams is always to push you forward, encourage you to shift your mindset and *do* something positive in your waking life.

9. And on the subject of moving forward every evening, when you finish your dream decoding is the perfect time to set the intention for your next dream or ask your dreaming mind for help (*see Dreamscaping, aka dream incubation advice, on page 233*).

To help you see dream cure decoding guidelines in action, I will now outline how to apply them to the most commonly reported dream themes. Please be aware that I'm using the word 'common' here simply to refer to the frequency with which they are reported to sleep and dream researchers and not in the meaning of them being 'commonplace'. No dreams – even those that feature everyday themes – are commonplace.

They will always be extraordinary and unique in their expression of these themes to you.

However, I hope running through themes that are likely to occur and offering you suggestions on how to interpret them will give you a solid foundation to start decoding the healing wisdom of your own dreams.

You will notice that each dream theme has many possible interpretations – and there is plenty of room for more. The aim is to encourage you to consider a vast range of possibilities and to connect them to your own personal associations and what is currently happening in your waking life.

DREAM THEMES

The most commonly reported dream themes are, in alphabetical order:

BODY PARTS

If your dream highlights certain body parts, these will be likely to reflect your inner thoughts. Body language experts can tell a lot about a person's well-being by studying their body and the way they move. You can do the same for the body or bodies that appear in your dreams. Of course, rule out any health issues first and then go with your personal associations before exploring common interpretations.

To help you think along the right dream-decoding lines, here are some key words for any body parts that may be spotlighted in your dreams.

Head: The self, your persona; what you believe about yourself and present to the world; the direction you are headed in

Neck: Your flexibility and ability to see differing viewpoints

Hair: Strength and vitality

Ears: Your ability to listen and absorb

Eyes: The windows of your soul – what you want to see or do not want to see

Nose: Something or someone in your face, close to you, invading your inner world; what you are breathing in, absorbing

Throat: How you express yourself or speak up for yourself

Arms: Your ability to embrace life

Hands: What you can grasp, hold or let go of

Fingers: What is slipping through your fingers

Back: Your support system

Lungs and chest: What you take in and hold in your heart; also, what you give out

Breasts: Nurturing potential

Heart: Unconditional love

Stomach: New insights

Genitals: Feminine and masculine traits

Anus: What you release or need to release

Legs: Movement forward, back or sideways – momentum

Feet: What grounds you

Skin: What makes you unique, but also what covers and protects you

CHASED

In this commonly experienced dream, you find yourself being chased by a wild animal, a predator, a gang or a faceless stranger, and although you aren't sure why, you know they mean you harm, or even want to kill you.

In the great majority of cases, the monsters that chase you in dreams aren't literal, but this dream can sometimes represent the actual fear of being attacked, so, as always, do consider the literal interpretation and keep yourself safe. However, this dream is more likely to be a representation of issues you haven't dealt with or aren't dealing with in your waking life. This dream can be a good indicator of a fear that is making you feel you're on the run.

Your dreaming mind wants you to consider what triggers your desire to avoid, evade and run away. You may not be able to change anything in your waking life, but this dream will help you become aware of what is likely to undermine your self-confidence so that when those fears are triggered in your waking life, you can find positive ways to manage them. Running away isn't one of them. Ask yourself who or what is chasing you, as this will offer insight into the source of your fears.

Or is the dream suggesting that you aren't considering a certain viewpoint or idea? Is the attacker perhaps a self-destructive part of yourself – your own repressed feelings of anger, jealousy, and so on? Are you projecting those fears onto someone or something else?

If you are doing the chasing in the dream, this suggests you may be pinning your hopes on and investing your energy in someone or something that is proving elusive. Anytime you chase or try to force things in your waking life, you are coming from a position of lack. The message of this dream is to stop chasing and attract what you want instead.

CHEATING AND AFFAIRS

Dream affairs are exceedingly common. In most cases they have nothing to do with cheating or the desire to cheat in waking life, unless you or your partner are already thinking about or actually cheating.

Everyone has these dreams, even those who are in a committed relationship. It's entirely normal, because humans are curious beings, and in your dreams, you can safely explore relationship scenarios without hurting anyone. So, don't feel guilty. A dream like this doesn't mean that you want to cheat, but it does suggest you are cheating *yourself* out of something. Your task is to find out what that something is, and what that word 'cheating' means to you.

So, cheating dreams are most likely to be about your own psychological needs. That's why you may wake up with a hot dream about someone who actually gives you the ick in waking life. When that happens, the first word that comes to mind when you think about that person is key. That association is what your dreaming mind wants you to get more intimate with.

Perhaps it is some quality you need to be more intimate with or some aspect of yourself you are denying or something you need to discover within yourself. For example, if you don't fancy your colleague, but they have a great sense of humour and you tend to take life very seriously, your dreaming mind might plunge you into a bad romance with your colleague to encourage you to lighten up.

So, don't panic – your cheating dreams are rarely about the person you are dream-cheating with, they're all about amazing you and what you need to develop, understand, heal and embrace *within yourself* in order to evolve. Focus on the first word that comes to mind about the person you're having the dream affair with.

If you're cheating with a stranger, your dreaming mind is urging you to discover untapped creativity within you or to better understand your shadow side (*see page 205*).

If you are being cheated on in the dream, the meaning shifts slightly towards your relationships in waking life. If you are in a relationship, has your partner been preoccupied with work or a hobby, or have the two of you been neglecting spending quality time together? Or do you need to inject more adventure into your love life?

The personal and universal associations with 'cheating' are often interchangeable and you can safely assume that a dream with a cheating theme is all about exactly that – what are you cheating yourself out of? What are you feeling insecure about within yourself and in your waking life? What do you feel is missing and what new adventure or perspective will complete you?

CHEWING GUM

Dreams of chewing gum that you simply can't spit out are often connected to an experience that you want to move on from or leave behind, but keep mulling over. In general, things that you take into your mouth in dreams – dream food – represent communication issues and also what you need to process or integrate for your emotional and mental nourishment.

When you dream of chewing gum, something or someone in your waking life feels impossible to 'spit out'. Ask yourself if you have bitten off more than you can chew in some area of your waking life? Are you taking on too much? Are you the gum (glue) that keeps everything and everyone together? Or are you constantly beating yourself up for mistakes made in the past?

Whatever you are ruminating about or feel that you are stuck with in your waking life, your dreaming mind wants you to spit out what is no longer energizing or nourishing you.

DEATH AND DYING

Death and dying are a commonly reported dream theme and the optimum way to decode their meaning will be explored on page 210.

DROWNING

The literal interpretation can be easily dismissed here, unless you plan on going diving or swimming in deep water. If that is the case, do your safety checks diligently.

Let's move swiftly on to your personal response to that dream of drowning. Water is a potent symbol of emotion and the unconscious world. Is there an area of your life where you feel overwhelmed or out of your depth in some way? This could be a work stress or a relationship issue that is dragging you down emotionally, or something in your waking life that feels tough to process.

Now move to the more abstract or common associations with drowning and again apply them to your waking life. Are you losing yourself in something or someone? Is there a weight of expectation on you? In what area of your daily life are you struggling to breathe or keep your head up?

Return to the emotional theme of the dream, because that will be central. If it is panic, your dreaming mind is urging you to find ways to deal with what is overwhelming you, or to ask for help and support. If, however, you find that you can breathe underwater, this is a sign that you are finding ways to adapt and make a challenging situation work for you.

A variation of drowning dreams but with similar interpretations is dream tsunamis and tornados causing devastation. The symbolism of potential emotional turbulence or feelings of instability is clear. Think about what or who is pushing your boundaries right now, or are you yourself creating a storm? It is not untypical for people going through periods of dramatic change to have these kinds of turbulent dreams. They could also point to a wave of hidden emotions and be warning you that if you connect to it, it will stun you with its surprising creativity. Don't fear your dream tsunamis. They are trying to tell you that sometimes when you think things are falling apart, they may be falling into place.

The dream is spotlighting the fact that unexpected changes are disarming you emotionally and you don't know how to react, as the old ways of reacting aren't working for you anymore.

You are in the thick of things and there is nothing to be gained from denying their reality. Accept that this change is happening, but as storms always pass, remember nothing is forever. Stay calm and let things flow over you until you are ready to emerge and take control over your life again.

EXAMINATIONS

In this dream you may find yourself in an examination room or classroom, sitting at a desk with a paper in front of you. You have absolutely no idea why you are there or what the exam is about, or if you do know what the exam is about, you can't answer any of the questions.

Of course, if you are studying for an upcoming exam, this dream is helping you process your nerves. It can also be a gentle reminder to make sure you do know what is coming up in the exam and are as fully prepared as possible.

However, most examination dreams aren't to do with literal exams but metaphorical ones. Consider what personal test you are undergoing at the moment and in what area of your life you feel you are being judged or examined. This could be anything from winning the praise of parents, teachers or employers to impressing your friends. Pinpoint where you feel you need to make the grade. Your dreaming mind could be warning you to do your 'homework' or make sure you are as well prepared as possible.

Universal associations with the symbol of examinations point to the idea of our entire lives being a test. So this dream could be suggesting that you are too preoccupied with gaining the approval of others. Indeed, a sign of personal and spiritual maturity is losing your need to be validated or approved of by others and, along with that, your fear of failure.

You understand there is no such thing as failure, as long as you learn and grow from it. In the words of Einstein, 'Failure is success in progress.'

Your dreaming mind may also be trying to reassure you. It has taken you to the scenario of being totally unprepared for something important, but the fact is you woke up the next morning and nothing disastrous happened. So it may be telling you that however much you feel you have messed up, or however much you feel like an imposter, you have the inner resources to pull through. You just need to believe in yourself.

Reassuringly, the people who have this kind of dream are often the ones least likely to be unprepared for an exam or upcoming challenge; indeed, it could be said that this kind of dream is one many highly successful people have. It is a sign of high expectations and a gentle warning that career expectations are only admirable if they coincide with personal happiness.

FALLING

Falling dreams consistently appear as the most commonly reported dream, but in some cases this may not actually be a dream at all. When you dream of falling, it can sometimes be related to the natural process of falling asleep. As you drift off to sleep, your heart rate slows down and blood pressure drops. These physical changes can not only induce a sensation of falling, but also trigger tiny bodily movements which may unexpectedly startle you wide awake.

Assuming it isn't related to the process of falling asleep and you don't jerk yourself awake, the first approach to this dream is to consider whether it might be a literal warning of something you may not have noticed or forgotten about in your waking life. For instance, are the steps outside your front door safe or in need of repair? No harm in making sure.

In the vast majority of cases, falling dreams refer to some kind of symbolic fall that you feel is happening in your waking life. Go with the first association you have with that word 'fall'. What immediately comes to mind in the context of your current waking life? Are you concerned about an upcoming result or status report at school or work? Do you feel that you can't keep up or that you have let yourself down in some way? Or do you feel that you have no firm ground or that you don't have the support of others?

Once you have considered your gut reactions to that word 'fall', you might want to refer to more generic uses of the word, such as 'fall from grace' and 'pride before a fall', and don't assume there are only negative associations. You can 'fall in love'.

Perhaps you have been told that falling in a dream and hitting the bottom is an omen of death, but this couldn't be further from the truth. Countless people have hit rock bottom in a dream and lived to tell the tale. And many of those people say that hitting the bottom in a dream is a liberating experience – nothing horrible happens and the dream carries on. Perhaps your dreaming mind, like the inner therapist it is, is taking you to the worst-case scenario on purpose. If you can 'see' yourself coping with and surviving your worst fears in your dreams, then in your waking life you know you have been there before and lived to tell the tale.

Key to this dream's interpretation will be the feeling falling inspired in you in the dream and on waking. If you were terrified, you must identify what is triggering the fear of 'falling' in your waking life and find ways to support and catch yourself. However, if you felt relaxed and enjoyed the sensation of falling, your dreaming mind is encouraging you to relax and go with the flow.

FINDING SOMETHING VALUABLE

If you have a dream about finding a hidden treasure, or a secret room in your house, or wads of cash, or winning the lottery, enjoy it and feel grateful. You never know, it could be a portent of a literal gain, either financial or emotional. In 2022 I was contacted by YouTuber and filmmaker Timothy Schultz, who in 1999 won nearly 30 million dollars on the Powerball lottery. He got in touch to tell me that a few months before that life-changing win he had a dream he would win, and that dream played out. (If you want to listen to him tell his incredible story, tune in to Season 6, episode 4, of my *White Shores* podcasts.)

However, when it comes to personal and spiritual growth, your dreaming mind considers inner wealth far more valuable than any financial gain. So it is likely that this dream is pointing to a feeling of self-worth that is either currently happening or needs to happen for you to get moving again.

Indeed, forward momentum is what all your dreams nudge you towards. They know that the best way to help you find inner peace and balance – rather like riding a bicycle – is to keep you moving forwards, even if that isn't always the direction you intended to head in.

What inner riches do you need to discover right now to give your waking life more momentum? Examine the circumstances of your waking life and consider what area you urgently need to inject with some happiness-attracting self-belief. The other supporting symbols – such as the item you find, or the location, as well as the feeling tone of the dream – will also offer helpful clues.

FIRE

Assuming there are no fire safety hazards in your life, consider what the word 'fire' means to you. What is the first association that comes to mind? Is it passion or destruction?

Bring in some universal associations with the element of fire to see if they enhance your personal interpretation. Freud associated fire with the libido, whereas Jung associated it with intuition and personal transformation. Just as the alchemists used fire to transform base metal into gold, so fire is a symbol for personal growth. It destroys the old and brings in the new. It is the eternal flame in the temple of your soul.

Fire is the bringer of light and life. It is often considered the most fearsome and potent of the elements, with the ability to bring warmth and light and to cleanse and purify, but also to bring pain and devastation. This dual symbolism means that the feeling tone of the dream as well as the other details of the dream are once again key.

If you aren't afraid of the fire in your dream, this could suggest you are letting go of old attitudes or a phase in your life that no longer serves you to make ready for the new. If you are fearful, this could suggest being fearful of change. Is the fire in the dream out of control? Are you being a hot head? Are you burning up inside? A controlled fire could suggest inner peace, with a fireplace pointing to the heart of the home and feeling comfortable with yourself.

If the fire in your dream is put out by water, could this suggest cooling or calming energies are needed in your waking life? And if the flame is confined to a candle, it may suggest the need to manage your impulses.

FLYING

Flying dreams are often accompanied by a sense of exuberance and liberation, both within the dream and on waking. Cherish these flying without wings dreams when they occur, because the majority of dreams are anxiety themed to encourage us to problem-solve and deal with areas of our waking lives that are stunting our personal growth. Flying dreams, however, are reflecting on our ability to happily rise above and express ourselves freely.

Of course, flying dreams can't be decoded literally, because it is impossible to fly without wings. Whenever you dream of something that is simply impossible in waking life, you must focus on the emotion of the dream. If you feel great in your flying dream, your dreaming mind is celebrating a personal achievement, suggesting that you are or soon will be experiencing a high, and you should pause and savour that moment, because you deserve it.

However, if you feel anxious when you are flying, this is your dreaming mind gently but firmly telling you that whatever you are worried about in your waking life, the solution is to rise above and see the bigger picture. In other words, try a different perspective and don't take everything so personally. There are some things in life you can control – your reactions being the key here – but there are also some things you simply can't control – the reactions of others, for example, or global events.

The height and ease with which you fly in your dream matter. If you feel nervous about flying high, this can indicate a fear not of failure but of 'shining'. Your dreaming mind is using this symbol to encourage you to believe in yourself more.

Once you have mulled over your personal associations with the symbol of flying in the light of your waking circumstances, do the same with the more abstract associations. In some schools of dream analysis, flying is associated with sexual energy, so consider whether this interpretation applies to your waking life. It is also associated with out-of-body experiences – mystical transcendent states where the soul leaves the body and travels into spiritual realms. See what resonates for you personally here. Flying could simply be a spiritual reminder that you are not your thoughts or your feelings. You have the ability to choose your thoughts and feelings, so choose them wisely. You aren't free to soar until you can master your thoughts.

Finally, flying dreams can be a precursor to lucid dreaming, when you know you're dreaming when you're dreaming (*see page 244*).

HAIR FALLING OUT

Dream hair loss is typically a symbol of personal stress. The most likely interpretation will be concerns about your appearance or ability to cope with someone or something that is happening in your waking life. Cancer patients may dream of their hair falling out as a way of coming to terms with their diagnosis.

Again, reflect on your immediate associations with the symbol of hair. Chances are it will be associated with perceptions of beauty or the appearance of youth.

Then consider the universal symbolism of hair, dating back to ancient times, when hair was typically believed to be a sign of a person's virility and fertility.

Losing hair therefore suggests feeling disempowered in some way or personal concerns with self-image. Pay attention to how you feel about your hair falling out in the dream. If it doesn't bother you, this suggests that you are letting go of attitudes or situations that no longer serve you. If you feel anxiety or embarrassment, your dreaming mind is urging you to address the cause of your current stress and the reasons why you may feel powerless and unappealing in your waking life.

LATE

If you are someone who often arrives late, this dreaming of being late could be urging you to improve your waking time management. However, in most cases dreams about arriving late for an interview, appointment, flight, train or date, despite your best efforts to arrive on time, signify FOMO – fear of missing out on opportunities in your waking life.

Try to identify who or what makes you late in the dream. If you clock watch in the dream or feel overcome with fatigue, this is a sign that you may be in danger of burnout in your waking life. Ask yourself what you fear you are missing out on and who you feel is moving ahead of you and leaving you behind. And at the same time, ask yourself why this matters. Should it matter? The only person your dreaming mind wants you to compare yourself to or get ahead of is the person you were yesterday.

LOSS

In some cases, dreams which feature the theme of loss can reflect concerns about actual things you have lost or people you have lost contact with in your waking life. However, chances are your personal association with the symbol of 'loss' is losing something or someone that is valuable to you. So, perhaps your dreaming mind is urging you to appreciate the people and things you take for granted in your waking life?

More universal associations with the theme of loss you might want to consider point to 'loss of direction or purpose' or even 'loss of confidence'. According to Jungian analysis, dreams of being lost or losing something or someone valuable to you suggest forgotten aspects of yourself you need to reconnect with. Your personal association with whatever and whoever is lost in the dream will be key here, as will the feeling tone of the dream.

Many of us will experience dreams with themes of loss when we are going through times of stress. This stress can be triggered by fear of failing an upcoming exam or interview or a relationship breaking down. There are countless aspects of loss, from losing possessions or friends and loved ones to losing personal freedom and aspects of your own personality. Loss dreams are also common during bereavement, as the dreaming mind works to help you process the grief.

The circumstances of the dream will add to the meaning. Do you know why you have lost something? Are you yourself lost? Have you taken a wrong turning? That wrong turning may help you identify the cause or reason. Your dream may even be reminding you that being lost isn't a crime. You have to be lost before you can find yourself. Remember, 'all who wander are not lost', to quote the wisdom of Tolkien.

However distressing or frustrating dreams of loss may feel on waking, please remember they are not meant to cause you anxiety. Your dreaming mind has conjured up these images to alert you to something significant and to help you cathartically release stress. As a rule of thumb, whenever a dream scenario causes you feelings of loss and sadness on waking, try to pinpoint what caused you the most tension in your dream. This may hold the key to understanding and healing the root of your fear.

Losing money, keys, phone or other valuables

Is there a literal interpretation? Perhaps you have misplaced the item you lost in your dream or your valuables aren't in a safe location and are at risk of being lost, so do a quick check.

Assuming they are secure, consider what the word 'valuable' truly means to you. Go as deep as you like and think about what your personal 'values' are and what you might be in danger of losing sight of. Bear in mind that one of the fastest ways to evolve is to get comfortable with 'letting go' and not holding on to things, relationships or mindsets that are no longer relevant or serving your best interests.

NUDITY

Always mindful of there being a rare literal interpretation, you might want to make sure there aren't any buttons or zips missing from your clothes! Assuming that isn't the case, this dream theme is indicating you may be feeling vulnerable or exposed in some way in your waking life. Also notice the reaction of others in your dream to your nudity. Chances are they won't notice or be bothered about it in the same way you are, suggesting you need to be less self-conscious as people are not judging or as interested in you as you think they are.

Dreams of nudity or being partially clothed don't typically have any connection to sex or anxiety about your sexuality, but are more about another area of your life being exposed or overshared. Your head may be convincing you that everything is okay, but your heart wants you to stop oversharing your opinions and comparing yourself and explaining yourself to others. This can put you in a vulnerable position. Save your explanations for yourself and focus on that relationship with yourself, on your strengths, not on what you lack. Over-reliance on social media for validation is often the trigger for nude or feeling exposed dream themes. The remedy? Limit your social media use.

This dream can feel alarming, but it is actually a very good sign, because it is only when you understand how vulnerable, how 'naked', you are that you can make changes in your waking life to protect your boundaries.

Dream nudity can connect to a longing to return to the innocence and spontaneity of childhood, or to show the world the real you. Perhaps you desire to rid yourself of pretence or a façade or living up to the expectations of others. In dreams, clothes conceal, protect and reveal, as they do in waking life, so this dream could be about the persona you have created for other people or the desire to be free of inhibitions in some way. How you feel about being naked in your dream is the biggest clue to how at ease you currently feel within yourself and how in harmony your head – what you think you should do – and your heart – what feels right to you – are.

OUT-OF-CONTROL CAR

From the messages sent to me over the years, a good many of my readers' dreams feature driving or being stuck in a car that is out of control.

Assuming there are no problems with your mode of transport, consider what personal associations you have with cars. If you own one, it is your personal space, your ticket to anywhere you decide to drive it. So, if in the dream your car is out of control or you can't get it to stop, or it's stuck or not functioning properly, think about how in control you feel of your life.

Pay special attention to whether you are driving the out-of-control vehicle or not. If you aren't driving, who is? You need to find out why someone else has taken control and what you need to do in your waking life to get back where you belong – in the driver's seat of your own life.

The universal interpretation of cars, trucks, bikes, planes, boats and any other mode of transport in a dream also suggests the direction your life is headed in. If you experience this dream, reflect deeply on the symbolism and speed of the mode of transport and what it suggests about where your waking life is currently headed.

PREGNANCY, GIVING BIRTH, A BABY

First of all, consider the obvious: are you pregnant in your waking life? I've had many messages from people over the years who have dreamed they're pregnant or known the gender of their child through symbols in a dream.

Assuming pregnancy isn't the case now, are you hoping to be pregnant, because if that is the case, this could be your dreaming mind preparing you for the role of parent.

If having children isn't a priority, consider what the symbolism of 'giving birth' or 'a baby' suggests to you personally and relate that to your waking life. Are you starting a new project or considering a fresh perspective, or does someone or something in your life (and that could be an idea) need nurturing, loving unconditionally and protecting like a baby? What new life within yourself are you giving birth to?

Now bring in some more generic associations with pregnancy. Something new is taking hold and patience is needed before the time is right for it to reveal itself to the world. What in your life is worth settling down and waiting for? Alternatively, is there something you want to 'give birth' to? This could be a new job or creative endeavour.

Or could this dream theme suggest that your own inner child, the part of you that is spontaneous, trusting and passionate, is in urgent need of more attention? Is it time for you to focus your waking energy on your own self-care and to give yourself unconditional self-love?

In summary, if pregnancy or a baby features in your night vision and you have ruled out any waking preoccupation with having a child, reflect on the personal symbolism of pregnancy to you – a new lease of life perhaps? Then consider whether the universal associations with babies resonate or add to your interpretation. Ask yourself what is happening in your waking life to inspire your dreaming mind to draw your attention to your own creative and/or nurturing feelings.

REST-ROOM

Closely related to dreams of being naked are dreams where you simply can't find a rest-room, and if you do find one, you can't use it or find that it is clogged.

Assuming there are no issues with the plumbing in your home or workplace, and you don't actually need to go to the toilet when you fall asleep, this dream is urging you to reflect on how well you are meeting your intimate emotional needs.

This common dream theme is highlighting the frustration you may feel when your privacy, boundaries or personal space is compromised, or if caring for others impedes your ability to care for yourself. Caregivers who constantly sacrifice their own well-being for others are prone to this kind of dream. Their dreaming mind wants to alert them to the importance of seeing to their own emotional needs first and to remind them this isn't selfish. It is the most unselfish thing, because you can't give to others what you can't give to yourself.

SNAKES

Assuming you aren't living in a climate where there are deadly snakes, this symbol stands out for the simple reason that snakes typically ignite an intense reaction in the dreamer.

Your personal associations are vital here, because if you aren't afraid of snakes, the more positive meaning of this symbol can apply. Snakes are potent symbols of transformation (they shed old skins) as well as stealth, mystery and endurance – they have thick skins and can survive against the odds. Snakes can also be symbols of healing and the harmonizing of two opposing forces.

However, for most people, snakes are evil predators and symbols of threat, so consider who or what in your waking life is alarming you or has the potential to intimidate you with poisonous words or deeds. And don't rule out the possibility that sometimes your own inner critic is the biggest threat. Whenever that inner critic surfaces symbolically in your dreams, try to show it compassion. It is likely to have evolved as a protection mechanism at some point in your life, so came with good intentions, but has simply outstayed its welcome. Thank it and then release it.

Once you have considered your personal associations with snakes, reflect on whether universal interpretations offer more illumination. According to Freud, there may be a sexual nuance, given that snakes are a phallic symbol, not to mention the kundalini snake is a sexual awakening, and according to Jung, snakes represent the mysterious part of the self. There is also an association with the afterlife, if you have lost a loved one. Bear in mind other associations, from 'a viper in your midst' – someone who appears friendly but is not – to the serpent in the Garden of Eden, bringing knowledge of the world, for a price.

SPIDERS

Unless you live in a climate where deadly spiders are a genuine risk, it is easy to dismiss the literal interpretation here and go straight for the personal associations.

So, what do spiders mean to you personally? Is there a fear factor when you dream of them? Do you wake up feeling terrified, as Ron Weasley did in *Harry Potter*, or trapped, like Frodo in Shelob's web in *Lord of the Rings*? Or are you a spider enthusiast, evoking *Charlotte's Web* and Spider-Man and believing a dream spider to be a creative and powerful sign? After all, there is little more intricate and ingenious than a spider's web spun from nothing but the spider itself.

If you're a fan of spiders, seeing them in your dreams will have a more empowering interpretation. If, however, spiders bother you and the web they weave to catch and poison their prey seems cruel rather than something they have to do to survive, your dreaming mind is using this symbol to alert you to something hanging over you in your waking life. Is there something or someone in your life that is making you feel trapped or helpless? A complicated relationship or a stressful job, perhaps? Or is there an aspect of yourself, a negative mindset or toxic habit, that is scaring you? What fears are invading your life? Spiders are also associated with manipulation, so might point to deceit.

Once you have reflected on your immediate personal associations with spiders, it might be worth considering the cultural associations. These are often contradictory, with spiders representing dark mystery as well as ingenuity. Given their incredible ability to weave perfectly constructed webs, they're also respected as creators, and therefore represent divine feminine energy as well as innovation.

Is there a feminine energy or person in your life right now that is overpowering you? According to Freud, spiders are symbols of the mother or the controlling aspects of her you may unconsciously still fear.

Jung believed spiders represented the archetypal shadow or undesirable side lurking within us all. Modern dream theorists put a more positive spin on spider dream interpretation and reference the infinite calm, patience, resilience, speed and creative skill of spiders, and the helpful role they play in home pest control. It's also worth flagging that these strange little creatures that most of us loathe sharing our homes with are likely to be more afraid of us than we are of them, so if they appear in a dream, we may be exaggerating or getting things out of proportion in our waking lives.

Lastly, when it comes to dreams about spiders, size matters. The bigger your dream spider, the bigger the spider-like energy looming over your waking life, wanting you to react and make a change. Time to confront your fears head on. Activate your spidey sense (aka intuition) and do something about it quickly, before it consumes you. This is especially the case if you have recurring dreams about spiders.

Your dreaming mind is using this wicked but wonderful symbol to get you to pay closer attention to something unresolved or which you need to face in your waking life. That could be a worry, or a conflicted situation, or a relationship. Or it could be your own spectacular creative potential just waiting for you to unleash it. It's your spider dream and your life – you get to decide.

TEETH FALLING OUT

In this dream, your teeth crumble or fall out one by one and you may feel helpless and embarrassed. Or you may dream of your teeth rotting or gums swelling with infection.

Consider whether you are due for a dental check-up. Your dreaming mind could simply be urging you to pay closer attention to your teeth and gum health, as the health of your teeth can be a good indicator of the health of your heart.

If your teeth are in good health, reflect on your own personal associations with teeth. What emotion would the symbol of a missing tooth inspire in you? Most likely it would be an assault to your self-image, a sign of weakness or vulnerability. Have you 'lost face' in some way in your waking life?

At this point, if the dream message isn't yet clear, you can also start to consider more universal associations with missing teeth. In the animal world, teeth are powerful ways for animals to communicate or to assert themselves. So, have you not expressed your true feelings in your waking life? Have you not been assertive or decisive enough recently? In what area of your life have you been toothless?

Being toothless is also considered unattractive, so are you overly concerned about your appearance or struggling to adjust to signs of ageing, as losing teeth tends to happen in old age? However, losing your milk teeth is also a wonderful sign of growing up, so this dream could also be all about the importance of letting one phase of your life go and moving forward with greater confidence into the next. Are you leaving school, moving house or starting a new job or role in your waking life?

To recap, if you have the very common dream of teeth falling out and have no problems with your teeth in your waking life, reflect on the symbolism of teeth to you – associations with appearance, issues with communication. What have you said or wished you had said?

Then consider whether any universal associations with teeth offer helpful new perspectives. Ask yourself what is happening in your waking life to make you feel 'toothless' or unassertive in some way. Do you feel disillusioned or are you feeling the emotional cost of making a compromise to keep the peace or stay on track?

It is through the gaps or the cracks (in your dream teeth) that the light will come in. What perspective shift or practical steps do you need to make in your waking life to protect yourself from the inside out? More often than not, when you have this recurring dream, your dreaming mind is urging you to reassess your priorities and make your own well-being top of the list.

INSTANT DREAM DECODING

There's been a lot to take in with this overview of common dream themes, so let's take a moment to pause, reflect and regroup.

I hope you have been recording your dreams and are getting close to harvesting a captivating series of at least 20 dreams. Right now would be the ideal time to review those dreams and see if you can identify any of the common dreams or variations of them that are mentioned above. Whether you can identify any or not, here's a snapshot reminder of the best way to start decoding your dreams:

- Eliminate the very rare possibility of a literal interpretation.

- Consider your immediate personal associations with key symbols or themes.

- See if universal meanings bring additional illumination.

- Identity the feeling tone of the dream.

- Wait for that 'Aha!' moment of uplifting clarity, and if it doesn't come, relax and dream another dream.

ASKING QUESTIONS

You will have noticed that asking your dream questions is the foundation stone of interpretation. Of course it is. Questions are infinitely more powerful than answers when it comes to personal growth, because questions encourage you to stretch your mind and seek out new possibilities. Answers do the opposite: they make you settle. Your dreams want to keep you moving, so they will form a big question mark in your mind every night.

Don't fret if you can't always answer the questions a dream asks of you. Sometimes the asking is enough to stimulate your creativity and give you the momentum you need in your waking life.

Never stop asking your dreams questions, because asking questions means you are open to new perspectives and ready to move out of your comfort zone, and outside your comfort zone is where meaning and adventure are found.

That's why it's a good idea to close every dream-decoding session in your dream journal with one more ongoing question:

Start that question with the words 'In coming days' and keep the focus on asking what more you can do to heal from the inside out. There will always be more you can do. Listen to that song from *The Greatest Showman*, 'Never Enough'. If your dreaming mind had an anthem it wanted you to hear, that would be it.

For example, if you've dreamed of losing your teeth, ask yourself:

'In coming days, when I feel I am losing face, what do I need to do to heal from that feeling?'

Or if you've dreamed of being drowned:

'In coming days, when I feel I'm not coping, what can I do to protect myself?'

'In coming days, what can I do to better prepare myself for an upcoming challenge?'

Or if you've dreamed you were in a car accident:

'In coming days, what can I do to feel more in control of the direction my life is headed in?'

Leaving your dream-decoding session in this open-ended way will underline to yourself that you are fully aware your dreams are your inner therapist. You know they want to encourage you to change your life in some positive way.

A LITTLE NIGHT POETRY

In all the common dream themes discussed above, you can see how your dreaming mind has created a visual story or image to convey a message to you about your mindset and/or the way you're currently handling a waking situation. As mentioned at the start of this lesson, it does this by using symbolic language in much the same way as a poet, novelist or artist would.

I'd like to take you back in time now to your English litera-ture class at school, when your teacher placed a poem in front of you. On first reading, you probably didn't have a clue what it meant and thought it sounded like nonsense, but then you were taught literary criticism techniques and the meaning became clearer. That's how I'd like you to approach your dreams from now on: as night poetry, eager to be interpreted.

If you dreaded poetry analysis at school and simply couldn't get your head around the idea that words can have many meanings and not just one definitive one, dream work is your second chance to take this on board. In fact, it's your chance to shine artistically. However logical you are in waking life, you are still wildly unpredictable in your dreams. Within that unpredictability lies the creativity of your inner artist and poet. Interpreting your dreams can directly connect you to stores of creativity you didn't realize you had. Give your dreams a chance to prove to you that there is method in their madness and a poet lives in you.

Poetry analysis techniques can provide a method to work with and give a dream the enticing feel of a cryptic crossword just waiting to be solved. They can help you transform what appears to be illogical nonsense into something that makes sense for you.

So, in addition to brainstorming the symbols, when you start decoding, ask yourself if your dreaming mind is using any of the following:

- *Simile:* Comparing one thing to another; for example, if a mouse appears in your dream, does this suggest panic or the need for silence, as in 'as quiet as a mouse'?

- *Metaphor:* Referencing one thing by mentioning another; for example, if gold appears in your dream, does this suggest wealth or 'a heart of gold'?

- *Personification:* Giving non-human objects or concepts human characteristics; for example, if a talking teapot appears in your dream, what is brewing in your life?

- *Sensory:* Consider how your dream appeals to your senses of touch, taste, hearing, smell and sight. In your waking life, pay attention to those senses more.

- *Pathetic fallacy:* The natural world mirroring the trauma of the central character is a literary technique often used in poems and novels to add intensity; for example, thunderstorms when heartbreak strikes. Your dreaming mind loves to use settings in this way too.

🌀 *The voice or viewpoint:* Is it in the first or third person? Are you experiencing what unfolds in the dream or observing it? If you are the observer, is your dreaming mind trying to encourage you to see the bigger picture and consider other perspectives? Or, depending on how you feel witnessing the action, does your dreaming mind want you to get more involved?

Other figurative language techniques to ponder are your dreaming mind's love of word play, hyperbole and puns. This may surprise you, but your dreaming mind really does have a sense of humour. Sometimes it will speak to you like a cartoonist. For example, if someone is bugging you in your waking life, it may well send you a dream about insects crawling all over you.

Another dimension to add to your dream interpretation is the dream use of idioms, expressions and slang, and also body language. And just as you would with a poem or work of art, always consider the overall feeling tone or mood of the dream, as that will speak volumes about the meaning.

One way to identify all of this artistic licence is to read your dream out loud after writing it down, or, better still, to try drawing it and to give it a title or caption. Your ability to do this will not only enhance your dream decoding, but also connect you to a deeply artistic, ironic, witty part of yourself that you may not have realized you had.

If your dream was a movie or book, what would be the underlying message or purpose of that movie or book?

LIVE THE DREAM

You'll know when you are on the right lines with your dream decoding, as you'll feel energized and uplifted. Any interpretation that drains or diminishes you isn't the correct one, because dreams are messages from your higher self. They want what is best for you, even if that sometimes makes you feel uncomfortable.

You will also get an 'Aha!' moment. If you reflect on all the associations at once, sometimes that Eureka moment will suddenly come. Other times it will jump out from nowhere when you aren't actually thinking about the dream. This is because routine tasks keep your conscious mind preoccupied and on autopilot, leaving your dreaming mind free from the restraints of logic and reason.

This is also what happens when you walk in nature or listen to music or absorb yourself in a task you love. All these activities distract your conscious mind and give your dreaming mind a chance to make brainstorming connections and call out to you. So sometimes it is a matter of simply trusting that dream-decoding revelation will come.

One way I love to trigger that revelation is to – within reason, as health and safety always come first – live or act out parts of the dream. Doing this is a super-powerful way to reassure your dreaming mind that you are taking it seriously. For example, if someone appears in your dream that you haven't heard from for a while, text them to ask them how they are and see what they reply. Or if your dream placed you in a park, seek out your local park. Or if you dreamed about a pack of lions watch a documentary about lions, and so on. The idea is that recreating an element of the dream will trigger a revelation. So, try to find a way of bringing safe elements of your dreams into your day. (Your dream journal template will include a reminder for you to do this every day.)

SEE YOUR OWN NIGHT LIGHT

Hopefully by now you will be starting to see your own inner light – or should I say 'night light' – when it comes to approaching common dream themes and relating them to events or thoughts in your waking life. The next lesson will be about more frequently reported dream scenarios and how you can expect those to alter during the different ages and stages of your life.

However, just before you do that it is important to discuss those *exceedingly* rare occasions when your dreams aren't symbolic but literal. Then I'll offer you a few more interpretation pointers to consider.

LITERAL OR SYMBOLIC?

You will have noticed that when discussing dream themes and how to decode them, I asked you to swiftly dismiss the literal interpretation first. I'd like you to continue to do that, because it will keep you on your toes and remind you that your dreams are a wildly mysterious force that can't ever be fully tamed or defined.

What is known is that your dreams are always trying to get you to look within yourself for answers. The majority of times they do that by symbolizing your mindset, but every so often, to stop you becoming complacent and to keep your mind open with questions, they do resort to the literal.

In some dreams, you encounter people and things you are familiar with in waking reality or as you go about your day as normal. What do these dreams mean?

If a dream character is someone or something you encounter regularly or daily in your waking life, this dream could be referring to that person or thing, but it will still use the language of symbols to do so.

Jung asserted that dreams about people we know intimately – loved ones and family – should be interpreted objectively rather than subjectively. Yes, in most cases we dream about our own mindset or internal world, but sometimes we dream about the nature of our relationships with others and what is going on for them or in the external world. Your personal reaction is again key. That is where the answer always lies.

To start sensing or knowing when a dream is symbolic and when it might be literal, record your dreams and with hindsight start looking for meaningful patterns. When you feel a dream is literal, take note of the symbols, themes and feel of that dream and if it played out in waking life. The more dreams you collect, the more you will notice similarities and instinctively come to understand when your dreaming mind is talking to you literally or figuratively.

WATCH YOUR ATTITUDE

I can't interpret your dreams for you. You are the only person who can do that. All I can do is offer you guidelines, but even if you diligently apply those guidelines, there will still be dreams whose meanings elude you. This shouldn't alarm you, because dreams are part of the enduring mystery of being human. Just keep on recording your dreams, linking them to events and thoughts in your day and becoming familiar with returning themes and their meanings for you.

Viewing all your dreams as a hidden treasure trove of self-realization rather than a life planner can really help you grow in confidence with your dream interpretation. And the more confident you become about your dream interpretation, the more confident you will become about your ability to cope positively and make better decisions in your waking life. I have seen people grow dramatically in self-esteem when they start doing dream work with me. It's a beautiful thing.

It may not have escaped your attention that many of your dreams try to tell you that much of your waking anxiety is self-imposed. Perhaps you fear not living up to the expectations of others or perhaps you expect the impossible, i.e. to achieve perfection. Or perhaps you are refusing to acknowledge your hidden fears or are applying out-dated coping strategies to new situations.

In these cases, it is your response rather than the situation itself that needs to change, and your dream is urging you to make that change so, moving forward, you can look at things more honestly or from a fresh perspective or simply draw on your own inner strengths. Your dreaming mind loves to point you towards your own mindset and how changing that can change almost everything.

CHILDISH THINGS?

The Jesuit saying 'Give me a child until the age of seven and I will give you the adult' is true to a certain extent, because how you were raised will shape how your brain develops and the kind of person you become.

It can be tough to escape early conditioning, but this doesn't mean it is impossible. Research shows that you continue to reshape your brain your entire life. The scientific term is neuroplasticity, meaning every time you learn something new, your brain changes physically, and it continues to be moulded by learning and experience throughout your life.

In other words, you can recalibrate old patterns at any time in your life. It won't happen overnight, but with dedication and passion, you can do it.

One of the best ways to release yourself from the limiting energy of negative mindsets you have inherited is dream work. Through your dreams you get to meet those limitations in symbolic form. Once you recognize what these symbols represent and how destructive it is for your inner world, in your waking life you can start consciously choosing different feelings, thoughts and actions. Keep repeating those positive feelings, thoughts and actions, and in time they will override any prior conditioning.

The best times to reshape your brain are just before you fall asleep at night and first thing on waking. This is because during those times your brain resembles the child-like impressionable state. You aren't fully awake and neither are you asleep. You are in a theta brain-wave twilight zone of suggestibility. In those precious moments, as well as telling yourself you will recall your amazing dreams, tell yourself that good things are coming your way and you are always good enough.

And if you wake up feeling anxious or negative, take a deep breath. This happens to us all at times. In ancient times, waking up paranoid was a potential life-saver, as falling asleep put you in a position of vulnerability, so it is possible that our brains are naturally hardwired to wake up on the anxious side. Knowing that, be compassionate towards yourself and choose to redirect your thoughts and feel energized instead.

SOMETHING ALWAYS COMES ALONG

If the meaning of a dream continues to be elusive, you can decide to let it go and dream another dream (there are always plenty more where that one came from) or you can continue to contemplate the meaning. If you choose the latter, you might just find that the more you consider all the possible associations and keep that dream on your mind, the closer you'll get to an interpretation.

Whenever I have a dream that I can't work out, I like to find somewhere quiet and safe to lie down and reflect on it during the day for a few minutes. I recall the dream and ask my intuition to send me a word, symbol, scene or image to help me understand it better. To paraphrase the dream wisdom of Jung, if you meditate on the meaning of a dream long enough, 'something almost always comes of it'.

As well as meditating on your dream, before you go to sleep you can ask your dreaming mind to bring you greater clarity in dream form. More about the life-changing potential of asking your dreaming mind for help in Lesson 5.

DREAMING ON

It is important to keep nourishing the creative and intuitive part of your brain so dream decoding starts to feel more instinctive, and that is precisely what Lesson 3 aims to do. It will examine scenarios your dreaming mind simply can't resist revisiting and exploring over and over again through the different stages of your life.

Just before you begin this lesson, take a moment to reflect on the following quote. Perhaps read it out loud. Notice with excitement the familiar and unfamiliar feelings it stirs within you.

A dream is not reality, but who's to say which is which?

The Mad Hatter

Then revisit the dream-work power points on page 4.

And now, dream on...

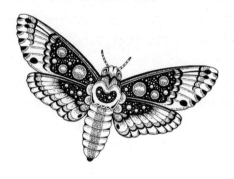

YOUR LIFE IN YOUR DREAMS

Night light: Your dreams surprise you into truly understanding that the definition of stupidity, to quote Einstein, is to do the same thing again and again and expect a different result.

That dream again!

Once you start consistently keeping a dream journal and start looking at it in hindsight, you'll be likely to notice repetition. Recurring symbols are common and highlight issues that you are facing in your waking life and how you are reacting to those issues. Their purpose, as with every single dream, is to help you process what is unsettling you and offer you opportunities to understand yourself better and find meaning and healing from the inside out. Typically, once you have understood the message of a recurring dream theme, it won't return.

YOUR DREAMING LIFE

Some repeating dreams are more common during particular stages in life, and they seem to coincide with the typical challenges of that stage. Of course, the following recurring dreams can happen at any stage in life, but here are some intriguing dream trends specific to certain life stages that I have picked up on in my decades of research. I'm confident that what you read for each stage of your life so far will resonate deeply with you.

CHILDHOOD DREAMING

Childhood is the time when you are most likely to have experienced vivid, intense and, at times, lucid dreams. Lucid dreaming (*see page 244*) is knowing you are dreaming when you are dreaming. It happens most frequently in childhood because children are less likely to question or fear it and simply enjoy the experience.

Recurring dreams in childhood are likely to incorporate terrifying elements, such as monsters under the bed or something scary chasing you. These dreams symbolize – as they continue to do if they return in adult life – feelings of not being in control of your life, which is, of course, the case for children.

Be aware that symbols that are frightening for children can represent the unpredictable side of their parents, carers, teachers and friends – the times when parents are stressed and snap or when teachers get cross or siblings bully. The dream is dramatizing how unsettling it can be when adults show a different face from the one a child expects.

Monster dreams tend to comment on parent and close family dynamics, with dreams of wild animals attacking becoming more common when a child starts going to school.

Another recurring sinister theme in childhood is toys or familiar objects suddenly coming to life and harming the dreamer. This often points to a fear of normal things in their life becoming unpredictable, as is the case when a new sibling is born or when a child starts a new school, and so on.

If you are a parent and your child wakes up with monsters, wild animals and other scary things on their mind, I urge you not to tell them it was 'just a dream', because this can seem as if you're saying that their anxiety isn't real, and discourage them from sharing their dreams (imagination, creativity) with you in the future.

Instead, ask them to describe their dreams, and don't judge or comment, just listen carefully. Sometimes just listening to your child talk about their frightening dreams is all the help they need. But if you detect a serious concern or trauma is triggering these dreams, be sure to consult a doctor or therapist.

Encourage your child to rescript any terrifying dreams so that the threat is disarmed. Ask them to narrate their dream and then change the ending so the monsters transform into butterflies. This will help them understand that they are the creator of their dreams and that nothing that happens in their dreams can harm them.

As a child matures, recurring dream themes may involve scenarios that are more task orientated, with the child dreaming of being required to perform unpleasant tasks against their will. This highlights their uncertainty about becoming part of a system they have little say in.

Drowning dreams are also common, and suggest feeling thrust into a situation without the emotional resources to cope or 'keep your head above water'. This dream can resurface in adulthood whenever you feel you are too deep into a situation and feel emotionally overwhelmed, so look out for it and reflect on whether the lesson it tried to teach you in childhood has been learned.

Other recurring dreams during childhood reflect the optimism and excitement of youth. Superhero themes – where the dreamer suddenly develops superhero powers and saves the world in the process – showcase the child's desire to discover within themselves the courage to make all their problems vanish. And flying dreams indicate the discovery of hidden talents and the desire to break out, to be independent.

TEENAGE DREAMING

The teenage years are often dramatic and confusing, as a child's search for identity takes centre-stage. Recurring dreams during this time reflect this intensity, with themes that dramatize the end of one era and the beginning of another. Dreams of death and dying, funerals and burial are common. Often those dreams involve the death of a parent and teenagers may wake up feeling anxious it's a premonition or that they unconsciously desire the death of a parent. Neither is usually the case.

Dreaming about the death of a parent at this time is simply a commentary on the end of one phase in a parent–child relationship and the beginning of another. This dream theme may reoccur when the time comes to go to college or work, leave home, get married, and so on.

Another recurring dream motif at this developmental stage may be of being aware you have killed someone and the body needs to be disposed of. This is a potent symbol of aspects of yourself that you feel you need to grow out of or dispose of. Watch out if burying-a-dead-body dreams return in your adult life – this could be a sign that you need to reconnect with the childlike parts of yourself that you should never have 'buried' in the first place.

A teenager's desire to belong and feel validated by others may also surface in dreams of meeting celebrities or famous people. Taking note of who those celebrities are could indicate areas of the teenager's life in which they long to excel or make their mark, or talents they have that are waiting to be noticed. Those celebrity-theme dreams may well happen in other developmental stages of life, too, when your dreaming mind wants to reference your desire for attention.

Whatever age you are, if you do find that a celebrity or famous person pops up in your dreams, whether repeated or not, it is well worth spending time researching that person. Read their biography. Consider the challenges they faced and how they dealt with them. There could be lessons and a wealth of personal growth insight waiting for you to discover there.

ADULT DREAMING

As you enter your twenties and thirties, recurring dream themes tend to reflect the frenzy of starting a career, finding a life partner, starting a family and all the traditional expectations that you may or may not feel you need to conform to. Not surprisingly, themes of running late, missing flights, being unprepared at work, failing an exam, forgetting lines on a stage and familiar routines or tasks suddenly becoming impossible to complete are common.

These recurring dreams all reflect a sense of frustration that although you have tried to do the right thing, you may have made the wrong decision, that opportunities have been lost or that you haven't worked hard enough or ticked all the boxes in time. Or that you simply aren't good enough.

If a recurring dream features tasks that you know you can do with ease, such as making a cup of tea, suddenly becoming impossible, this references your approach to a current situation. You are approaching a problem in the old way when what you need to do is find a new way. In other words, you need to change your strategy.

The familiar-suddenly-becoming-unfamiliar theme is urging you to not just find new approaches, but also to stop comparing your performance to that of others. In the dream you may feel deeply embarrassed you can't get easy things right, but the reality is nobody is judging you harshly but yourself.

Your inner wisdom knows that your search for perfection is your biggest roadblock, as perfection is impossible, and not even desirable, as it leaves no room for improvement or learning and growth.

Interestingly, imposter-syndrome dreams, such as forgetting lines on stage or not being up to an important task at work, typically happen to people who are high-achievers and who in waking life won't allow themselves to fail or be late or unprepared. However, the dreaming mind in its infinite wisdom knows that failure is important for personal growth, so it forces a person to dream about experiencing failure so they learn from it from within.

Of these frustrating recurring dreams where you don't feel you are on top of things, the missed flight or train theme is perhaps most likely to recur, as it is the dreaming mind's way of gently reminding you that in your eagerness to press ahead, you may be forgetting to pay enough attention to who or what truly matters in your life.

Another sign of potential overload and an overly busy life is a dream about losing or forgetting about a child or loved one and then panicking that you can't find them. This dream is a clear warning not to let the small stuff – the details in your waking life – get in the way of the big stuff. Have the demands of your schedule taken over your life and minimized the amount of quality time you can spend taking care of yourself and being there for loved ones?

Whatever age you are when you dream of missing flights or losing loved ones, be sure to take a moment to reflect on whether you are taking on too much in your waking life or if your perfectionist mindset is bringing you joy. Have you focused so much on a specific life goal or destination that you have forgotten to enjoy the process, the journey?

Watch out, too, for recurring dreams that take you right back to school or college, where you are unprepared for an exam or unable to gain entry to a college course. These dreams are all about your identity and are typically related to your sense of status in life and feelings of insecurity surrounding that. They are reminders that it doesn't matter how much you achieve or how high you fly in your career or how popular you are, without the inner foundations of self-love and self-belief, you'll forever feel that you are not quite good enough.

Bear in mind too that one of the most healing functions of dreams is to release stress by playing out behind your eyes the worst possible scenario. Knowing that you can cope with the worst-case scenario – because you have been there before in a dream – and that you should never let your entire happiness and sense of self be determined by any external event or situation, whether it is a success or not, is the key to unlocking the meaning of this dream.

As immortalized in Kipling's poem 'If', when you learn to rise above and not have your happiness determined by externals, when you can treat triumph and disaster, those imposters, both the same, then you are truly growing up.

MIDLIFE DREAMING

Recurring dreams from your mid-forties onwards tend to shift from anxiety themes related to the progress you feel you should be making to reflecting anxiously on whether the things you are doing are actually bringing you fulfilment.

One very common dream in this life stage is not being able to find your car or bike or other mode of transport, and trying to pretend to others that nothing is wrong. If you experience this dream theme, your dreaming mind is urging you to consider your accomplishments so far and to ask yourself what is missing from your life. What do you need to change to find satisfaction and deeper meaning? This could be your job, location, relationship or simply your mindset and the way you approach your daily life.

Pregnancy and baby-related dreams are also common during midlife, in particular the dream of hearing screaming and finding an abandoned baby. The baby in the dream is a clear symbol of a neglected inner child and/or some hidden potential or creative aspect of yourself or an interest or idea that has been neglected or put on the back burner.

You may also notice recurring dreams about everyday objects suddenly developing magical powers, such as a mug that can fly or a coat that can talk. This dream is not only spotlighting feelings of not fitting in or being an outsider, but also reminding you that often we look for excitement in exotic places, when the real treasure is in the ordinary.

Another recurring dream may involve themes of rejection by those you love or work with and everything going wrong and the hurt and confused feelings that accompany these disappointments. You may find you continue to have these kinds of unpleasant dreams until you change your attitude in waking life. Only when you understand that failure is the only way to learn, that rejection is an opportunity to course correct and that negativity is a personal choice will these kinds of dreams cease.

Similarly, recurring dreams of overcoming seemingly insurmountable obstacles and barriers, such as wading through mud, being locked in a dark room with no means of escape, being buried alive or screaming but not making a sound, are also symbolic representations of your mindset and the importance of changing it. Should you have these painful dreams or feelings in waking life, a mindset shift is key. They are clear signs you are about to learn and grow, become wiser. Sometimes growth hurts, but evolution is exciting!

MATURE YEARS

Anxiety dreams related to fears about ageing and your health and relevance declining are typical in the later years of life.

Not surprisingly, one common recurring dream theme in this era is getting lost and being unable to find your way home. Every route you take seems to make you feel even more lost, and directions given to you by others just confuse matters further. In this dream, the symbol of getting home is regaining your sense of self, and the incorrect routes and directions are symbols of well-meaning advice from others. Your dreaming mind is urging you to trust your own instincts over those of others.

Losing a wallet, purse or bag with all your essentials in it is also a recurring dream theme here. This is reflecting fears about the difficult changes that later years can bring and feeling you don't have the inner resources to cope. You may have this dream after retirement or a bereavement or downsizing to a more age-appropriate home. The message is to trust and let go, take all the time you need to ground yourself and do things that give you a sense of inner security.

Another recurring dream during this life phase is your phone malfunctioning or not working. Perhaps you are trying to get through to someone but you can't make the connection. Phones in dreams are classic signs of communication, so consider if there is someone in your waking life that you need to get in touch with or convey a message to, but more often than not dream phones are symbols of your own inner voice trying to send you an important message. And that message is that it is more important than ever to be as honest with yourself as you can, to ask for help if you need it and to talk compassionately to yourself.

HOLDING YOUR HAND

Despite the Hollywood cliché, recurring dreams aren't typically indicators of buried trauma; they are far more likely to be signposts, pointing you in a more positive direction. They tend to happen more during certain life stages than others and also rise to the surface during times of significant change or personal crisis, such as leaving home or going through divorce or bereavement, when you need to develop new coping skills and mindsets but don't know how.

Dreaming about emotional changes that are difficult to adapt to and process is cathartic and actually helps us cope better. This is certainly the case following bereavement, with those who say they dream of a departed loved one being better able to move through and beyond their grief.

Recurring dreams help by making associations that can point you towards healing. If you are going through a personal crisis and having anxiety-themed recurring dreams, this doesn't mean you are out of your depth; it means your inner therapist is working diligently to help you process and adapt. It is holding your hand.

However, it is always recommended that during times of painful life crisis you seek support and advice from trusted family members and/or a doctor or therapist.

LET IT GO

The longer you keep a dream journal, the easier it becomes to identify recurring themes, characters, locations and objects. You can also observe just how long your dreaming mind has been patiently trying to draw your attention to something in your waking life or your mindset which isn't in your best interests.

Identifying a recurring symbol or theme in your dreams can be a revelation, because when you spot it, you discover what your current roadblock to happiness is. And in almost all cases, the feeling tone of anxiety that accompanies the dream will be reminding you that you can't move past this roadblock until you allow yourself to think, feel and react *differently*.

Many of us cling to ways of thinking, feeling and reacting that may have felt relevant at one point in our lives, but as we age are no longer appropriate and may even have become toxic. A recurring dream is our nocturnal intuition telling us that things can only shift in a more positive and healing direction if we change our perspective.

Often recurring dreams spotlight attitudes or negative self-talk that have become so deeply ingrained that we have forgotten we actually have a choice about them. Sometimes it isn't easy to immediately choose a positive mindset. Observing a recurring dream offers you an opportunity to cruise in neutral or to decompress before rising from negative depths to positive heights.

Chances are, the negative thought patterns and behaviours your dreams are bringing to your attention evolved to protect or help you during a time when you felt vulnerable and alone. They were born with good intentions, but you don't need their 'protection' anymore. Simply let them go, and as you do, thank them for what they have taught you about yourself. There is always wisdom to be found in your wounds.

When you understand that a recurring dream theme is highlighting a glitch in your own mindset and/or approach, more often than not that theme will disappear. However, as the meaning of life is found in constant learning, other recurring themes will replace it to ensure you are always reflecting on what motivates you at a deep level and reaching for other perspectives. Sometimes those perspectives won't give you all the answers, but they will bring you an awareness of personal choice, and with that will come a feeling of empowerment.

Having said that, if recurring themes are not as obvious as before, this suggests you are making great strides in your personal and spiritual growth. As you have learned, your dreams reflect your waking mindset, so a dawn chorus of ever-changing dreams that aren't stuck on a loop are an indicator that you are living life as it is meant to be lived – as a spontaneous adventure.

AND BACK AGAIN

Reading about the infinite things you are most likely to encounter in your dreams and potential ways to decode them reassures your dreaming mind that you're serious about understanding the meaning of your dreams. It will also prime your brain to send you incredible dreams tonight.

If you have a favourite song that you never tire of listening to because it always brings fresh inspiration, I'm hoping you'll find the upcoming condensation of the infinite potentials you are most likely to encounter in your dreams will never fail to illuminate you in the same way.

I suggest from now on, along with your dream journalling, you make this book, and especially this chapter, your go-to dream-inducing read before bedtime. It won't ever become tedious reading. Read it and reread it – it's the dream heart of this book, an expansive deep dive that can help you hold your own when it comes to interpreting the wild and wonderful ocean depths of your night vision.

What follows is a condensed map of the dream world of recurring symbols and themes that I sense you will be recalling and writing up in your dream journal in the coming days, weeks and years. The interpretations here are by no means set in stone, and as always, your personal associations are crucial. Some of what you read will revisit decoding insights previously shared, but these are insights so crucial and constantly relevant for your healing dream work that they can never ever be reinforced or restated enough.

It is entirely possible that the details of a dream you have may not be listed or mentioned here, or anywhere in this book. However, those details can find a thematic home in one of the following categories, and the dream-decoding advice given in that category will help you interpret them. For example, dreaming of a skiing accident would belong to the 'Accidents' category, even though there is no mention of skiing in that category, and dreaming about a zebra would belong to the 'Animals' category, even though zebras are not specifically mentioned in that category, and so on. That is why making associations and identifying the essence of a dream symbol is so crucial to understanding it.

Dream research is making great strides, but we still have so much more to learn. Your desire to learn is what gives everything momentum in both your waking and dream life. The fact that you are reading this book is proof of your desire to learn more and more about the meaning of your dreams. Celebrate and cherish that desire, because it's going to take you far.

And from now on, whenever you dream decode, try this little tip from me: *smile* and raise your eyebrows as you write. Your unconscious mind will notice and adore you for it!

YOUR DREAM WORLD MAP

ACCIDENTS

Accident dreams highlight fears and worries. It can feel as if your dreaming mind is urging you to take responsibility before there is a crisis. According to Freud, accidents in dreams, like slips of the tongue in waking life, can offer direct clues to our unconscious motivations. For Jung, accident dreams offer insights into unconscious fears, or could be symbolic recreations of past emotional trauma to help us revisit and process it and heal from it.

Another possible interpretation is that your unconscious has noticed something potentially dangerous that you haven't noticed in your waking life. This could be a reminder or a warning. For example, you may have met someone new and felt uncomfortable around them, but dismissed your gut instinct. Your dreaming mind may then send you a dream of a venomous snake to encourage you to always trust your gut instincts.

ACTION

Action-themed dreams in which you are the Indiana Jones or Lara Croft of your nocturnal adventures are thrilling to experience and suggest an exciting personal breakthrough in your waking life is either being made or needs to be made. Your dreaming mind is applauding your experimental instincts or suggesting that the way forward is to follow them. The Jungian archetype of the hero battling adversity to learn, mature and grow dominates this interpretation, and adventure-theme dreams always support you getting right out of your comfort zone.

Actions within dreams also point to hidden motivations and agendas and are associated with progress or how to best move forward in waking life. So, is the action speeding you up or slowing you down? Did you achieve your goal or reach your destination? What was the goal or destination? The answers to such questions will help you assess your progress and identify and overcome any obstacles in your waking life.

Jumping, running, racing and dancing themes are also related to the level of attainment you hope to achieve and your progress towards it to date.

AMBITION

Our ambitions, both overt and hidden, love to surface in symbolic disguise in dreams. According to Adler, dreams are an expression of our unconscious craving for power, a way of compensating for our shortcomings in waking life. For instance, if you can't stand up for yourself at work, you may dream of a wrecking ball demolishing your workplace.

Some dreams are pure wish-fulfilment, but ambition dreams are more likely to be progress reports offering pertinent observations and warnings of things that haven't been registered by your conscious mind. If you become aware of them through your dreams, they can help you achieve your goals.

If you find yourself being a superhero in your dreams, your dreaming mind is giving you a vote of confidence. The message is that if you work towards and believe in your goals, you can find ways to overcome roadblocks in your waking life.

AMPHIBIANS

Amphibians and reptiles are dream symbols with multiple interpretations, but in general they suggest danger or being cold-blooded (hearted), and also the energy of slow healing over time. Try to recall how they behaved in your dream, as this should help you identify which aspect the dream is spotlighting. And remember your personal associations are key.

ANIMALS

In dreams, the appearance of an animal indicates urges and desires that are instinctual, hidden or craving recognition. It can also represent a part of you that is instinctive and hard to control. And because we often assign human characteristics to animals in dreams, they may symbolize gut feelings about others we would be wise not to ignore. An attacking lion, for example, may depict how you feel about someone who is aggressive or it could shine a spotlight on your own hidden aggression needing to be expressed and released healthily.

According to Freud, all dream animals are symbols of unexpressed sexual and aggressive tendencies. Jung, however, argued that animals in dreams should be analysed individually according to the personal association the dreamer had with the animal. He also suggested that animals symbolized the higher self of the dreamer, the part of them that followed its own natural inner laws, and so, in this sense, they were a source of spiritual wisdom.

The best way to start decoding the meaning of animal-themed dreams is first of all to think about the way you feel about that specific animal in your waking life. For example, if you love dogs, a dream dog will be a symbol of loving companionship, but if you are afraid of dogs, it won't have that heartwarming association.

Focus on the feeling(s) that the animal inspires in you, but if no feelings emerge, enjoy researching the universal, archetypal, mythical or magical associations of that animal; for instance, a hare is associated with speed, a fox with cunning, and so on. Your dreaming mind may be using this symbol to alert you to your own or someone else's cunning. Reflecting on that aspect of yourself within the context of the dream should tell you whether you need to nurture and develop it, tame it or be on your guard against it.

And remember how much the dreaming mind loves punning. If you dream of a badger, are you feeling 'badgered' in some way?

Whatever they are, dream animals offer a priceless opportunity to connect with parts of yourself that are buried because at some point you felt uncomfortable about them. In general, though, when an animal appears in a dream, it is a potent sign that your unconscious is wide awake and speaking to you loud and clear. As you interpret your dream, never forget that your dream animal is expressing the drive within you to live your life authentically and spontaneously.

Animals can also signify instinctive responses, such as the urge to mate or protect your family, and so on. Whenever these instincts need to be understood, expressed or controlled in some way, animals can appear in your dreams to symbolize them.

By understanding your dream animals and the qualities they represent, you can approach your life in a more natural way. Bear in mind that there will be a difference in the way you interpret the meaning of wild and domesticated animals in your dreams. In general, domesticated animals and pets suggest urges which you have more control over and are less threatening to your desire to be in charge. Wild animals suggest urges which are more threatening to your ego, but if you can develop a working relationship with them, they offer incredible potential for personal and spiritual liberation.

ARCHETYPES

The 'collective unconscious' is the term Jung used to describe a sort of psychic storehouse common to the shared memory and experience of humanity. The contents of this storehouse are called archetypes; they are patterns and symbols that can be found within the unconscious of everyone. Many of these archetypes are familiar to us from myths, legends and fairy tales. For example, the archetype of the mother is a universal symbol of nurturing and we are familiar today with the super-hero and villain archetypes, showcased in movies like the Spider-Man or Batman series.

Jung believed dreams were attempts to guide the waking self and that the purpose of our lives was to understand, love, heal and integrate all aspects of ourselves. Dreams are our unconscious trying to communicate and find harmony with our conscious self. In waking life our unconscious self is hidden, but in dreams it is revealed. You are most likely to encounter archetypal figures in your dreams at transitional times in your life rather than stable ones. Change inevitably brings about self-reflection; for example, when leaving home, moving house, or starting a family or new job, and so on.

The first step when analysing an archetype, as with any dream symbol, is through personal reference. For example, a dream about a murderer may refer to your archetypal shadow, but could also reference an overbearing relative. The next step is to take into consideration the other images in the dream, as well as the feelings it generates.

You will rarely feel indifferent when an archetypal symbol appears in your dreams and your instinctive response will be crucial for the interpretation. Does the dream make you feel angry or sad, happy or frustrated? Never forget these images come from the depths of your unconscious and you need to discover why they have surfaced at this precise moment in time. There's always a reason.

Although Jung believed there was no limit to the number of archetypes, he thought most were linked to the following aspects that constitute our personality: the *anima* and *animus*, the ego, the persona and the shadow.

The *anima* and *animus* are the male and female archetypal roles that we feel we must play. Often these can be traditional ones with women feeling they must fulfil the archetypal role of homemaker and men feeling they must be the strong bread-winner, but these traditional archetypes no longer speak to everyone. The *anima* is the female energy present in the collective unconscious of men and the *animus* is the unconscious male energy present in the collective unconscious of women. The function of the *anima* and *animus* is to establish a good working relationship with their male/female counterpart.

If someone of the opposite sex appears in your dream and triggers deep feelings, you may want to consider if your dreaming mind is tuning into the energy of your inner *anima* or *animus*. Typically, the *anima* or *animus* will be personified as a single figure, such as a maiden or a crone or a prince or a wise old man. By introducing this figure, your dreaming mind is urging you to seek balance and strengthen your connection with the opposite male/female energy within you.

The ego or self-construct in your dreams is arguably the most significant and it typically shows up in the archetype of a child or baby, suggesting your inner vulnerability, spontaneity and potential that needs to be carefully nurtured. For a woman, your higher self may be presented in the form of a dream priestess, goddess, fairy godmother, princess or queen, and for a man it may appear as a king, priest, wise old man or prophet.

The persona represents your public image or the part of yourself you present to others by what you say, wear and look like. It is what you reveal to the world around you or the mask you wear. Bear in mind that your persona may present itself as a dream theme, for example in a dream of being naked or inappropriately dressed.

Last, but by no means least, if you dream of someone who is a stranger or if you encounter monsters, criminals, prostitutes, burglars, villains, and so on, your dreaming mind could be using archetypes to reveal to you your shadow side, the part of you that is unknown or feels unacceptable to you.

The shadow (*see page 205*) may not always be presented as an enemy in your dreams. It can often contain qualities that you need to better understand and will only become hostile if you continue to ignore or misunderstand them. Although you may think of the shadow as the toxic side of yourself, it is amoral – neither good nor bad, just like animals. An animal is capable of tender loving care of its young, but can also become a vicious killer. It doesn't choose to do either; it just does what it does. It is innocent, though from our human perspective it can appear cruel. In the same way, the shadow part of ourselves is the part of ourselves that helps us survive, but that we can't quite admit to.

ARTISTIC ENDEAVOURS

Whether you dream of composing a symphony, painting a masterpiece, singing in an opera, acting on stage, directing a movie or designing a scrapbook, any dream that presents you in the role of artist or creator is all about the creative and intuitive side of you and its desire to be expressed in waking life.

If you are a naturally artistic person, dreaming of being creative may be less significant than if you are not. But whether you are artistic in real life or not, these dreams are your imagination and creativity calling your name. Listen to them.

If your creative dream involves a stage, platform, studio or theatre, this can indicate a desire to be more visible or for more people to appreciate you. If there is an audience, are you performing or watching? If you are performing, it suggests that you are overly concerned with the approval of others. If you are in the audience, this could be a sign that you either need to get more involved in the action or that you need to be more objective about something playing out in real time.

And should you ever hear music in your dreams, know that many of the world's greatest musicians heard their greatest works while dreaming or immediately on waking. The song 'Yesterday', for example, emerged from the sound of a dream Paul McCartney had. He woke with the song fully formed in his mind, and after confirming with everyone that he had not heard it anywhere before, he described it as a 'magic thing'.

Your dream music may also reference how you are currently feeling in your waking life, as music and dreams speak the same language of emotion and spirit, so tune into how the sound makes you feel.

BIRDS

What sets birds apart is their ability to fly, rise above, see the bigger picture and escape the limitations of Earth. They are a universal symbol of transformation and progress towards fulfilment in life. Their association with the element of Air – itself associated with aspiration – means they are also a symbol of high-flying ambition and the quest for enlightenment.

In Greek mythology birds are divine messengers, so in psychological terms dream birds show that your unconscious is offering wisdom. 'Taking a bird's-eye view' means being objective.

Dream birds can also symbolize relationships – for example, if you dream of a magpie, is someone in your life stealing your energy? – but they are more likely to spotlight the urge for freedom, liberation and spiritual growth. If a bird appears in your dreams, ask yourself if a part of you wants to fly away, escape from pressure and feel free. Or is there a situation you need to rise above? Or is your dreaming mind referencing a flight of fancy, something you wish would happen in your waking life?

Your dreaming mind conjures up images of birds to reflect your attitude or a situation, so do consider the type of bird that appears in the dream and both your personal and the common associations with that bird. At all times, the condition and health of the bird matter, and if the bird is suffering in any way, or caged, this suggests frustration. A flock of birds can symbolize both yourself and the people closest to you, and if the bird is dead, this could suggest loss of purpose or problems constantly on your mind.

Bear in mind that birds are also symbols of the soul or the afterlife, and throughout the centuries they have been considered both good and bad omens, depending on the type of bird. Zero in on the colour and size of your dream bird, as these will add deeper meaning to the dream.

BIRTH

Dreams of giving birth can be anticipation of the real event, but in most cases have no connection to the biological process of reproduction and more to do with a sense of being reborn, of fresh beginnings and ideas coming to fruition. For Jung, birth dreams represented personal growth, new starts. And if a baby appears in the dream, chances are your inner child is in urgent need of your nurturing attention.

BODY

Dreams about the body or parts of the body occur for several reasons. The first is that it is possible your dreaming mind is alerting you to health concerns you may not be aware of yet, so do always rule that out. The second is that such dreams are reflections of your own feelings about your body or appearance. The third is that in a dream your body often reflects your lifestyle. So, if anything is broken or injured, what part of yourself is at risk or are you losing?

Psychologists call the process of giving up parts of yourself to please others 'fragmentation', and if this is done for co-dependent reasons, your dreaming mind might be sending you warning signals. For example, if you dream your limbs fall off, what portion of your potential is being lost as a result of the path you have chosen in waking life? This is another interpretation of those teeth-falling-out dreams. Your dreaming mind is asking you just how much you are willing to compromise and reminding you that what you are losing is irreplaceable.

Another pointer to help you interpret this dream is to think of body-related expressions, such as 'losing your head', 'losing your right arm', 'not having a leg to stand on', 'being able to stomach it', and so on. When you say those things, you aren't being literal but expressing an emotion, and that is exactly how dreams love to speak to you.

BUILDINGS

Buildings in dreams represent aspects of your personality or your 'self-constructions'. The upper floors represent the conscious mind and the lower floors the unconscious. Different parts of a building may represent different times in your life and the attitudes and beliefs you have as a result of your experiences then. The features may mirror features of your personality, reflecting how you feel about yourself right now.

When a building appears in your dream, ask yourself what aspect of you does that building represent. Is it how you see yourself? If it is crumbling, are you in need of some kind of restoration? If it is burning, is this your desire to purge or release something you feel is holding you back? If it is in ruins, do you feel neglected or abandoned by others? If it is tall, does this suggest ambitions yet to be fulfilled? Ask yourself what the buildings in your dreams represent to you.

The condition of a building and the feeling it inspires will offer clues to its meaning, as will the purpose of the building in real life. For example, a castle is protection, a lighthouse is isolated but can also offer hope, a factory suggests work, a church offers reflection, libraries and museums supply knowledge, courts are about justice, prisons are about learning the consequences of your actions, hotels suggest a break from routine, airports and railway stations are about forward motion and getting on the right track, schools about learning, restaurants about nourishment, and so on.

CHANGE

It could be said that every dream has the theme of change, because change is an inescapable fact of life and your dreams always comment on or offer brainstorming solutions to what is happening in your waking life.

Dreams where obvious changes occur – for example, people, locations and objects transforming into someone or something else – suggest dramatic and immediate changes are required in your waking awareness. They can also represent unpredictable people or situations or emotions in your waking life, as well as new directions on the horizon or the need for a radically different perspective.

More subtle dream symbols which reflect change or the need for change in your waking life include dreams of yourself or others wearing disguises, dreams about goodbyes, of drifting in a rudderless boat, of clocks, of crossing a bridge, and mirrors with strange or no reflections. If you dream of being in a maze or labyrinth, this a powerful nod from your unconscious about the importance of finding inner direction and the skills to navigate change.

CHILDHOOD

It is in childhood that you develop your personality and learn about life, so if a dream takes you back to childhood, it will be focusing on lessons you learned or failed to learn then, and these lessons may be relevant to or repeating in your current waking life. This is especially the case if your dream takes you back to school (*see also page 180*).

CHILDREN

The symbol of a child references your own inner child, the part of you that is natural, curious, childlike and vulnerable.

If babies or children appear in your dreams, always apply their symbolism to your current circumstances. Do you need to learn how to play again or be adventurous, or does a part of you long to escape adult responsibilities? Or do the children represent a part of you that yearns to be nurtured and protected? They're your dream children. You decide.

CLIMBING

Any climbing or elevating theme in a dream suggests good progress towards your goals. What you climb signifies the scale of the task and how you climb comments on your tactics and whether they are helping or hindering your progress.

CLOTHES

In waking life, clothes protect, conceal and reveal, and so in dreams they depict the façade or persona you create for other people and tell you where you may be vulnerable or exposed in waking life. The colours, style and condition of the clothes are especially important, as they reveal how you feel about yourself or how others perceive you.

You may have the common dream of wearing the wrong outfit for an occasion or struggling to find clothes that are appropriate. This is all about your self-image and feeling vulnerable. Are you struggling to conform or fit in or do you want to free yourself from inhibition? The feeling tone of the dream will be key to the interpretation here.

If a dream spotlights a particular item of clothing, the key to its meaning will be the function of that clothing and your personal associations with it, as well as language associations. For example, if you dream of nightwear, this suggests the need for openness and relaxation, and if you dream of a hat, consider idioms such as 'changing hats' and 'drop of a hat'.

COLOURS

Your dreams may be crowded with colours, only for you to forget them on waking, and this is why some people believe they only dream in black and white. You may also think that the colours in your dreams are incidental to the main story and not pay attention to them. But the colours of your dreams offer vital clues to their meaning. I hope that from now on when your recall your dreams and write them up in your dream journal, you will be mindful of noting down their colours too. This will lead to a much richer and deeper interpretation.

For example, if you dream of a statue falling from a mantelpiece and crashing to the floor, you may focus on the statue falling, but if you note that the statue is green, a possible interpretation could be jealousy, as in 'green with envy'. So, could your dreaming mind be warning you about your or someone's jealousy and how it might sabotage a new relationship or project?

Colour affects our mood, because of the vibrational frequency each colour possesses. The colours in your dreams will tell you a huge amount about your emotional landscape.

Your dreaming mind chose a specific colour for a reason. Try to work out what your personal associations with that colour are and then explore the traditional or universal ones to see if they add more perspective. If you aren't sure what your associations are, one technique is to imagine you are describing a specific colour to a blind person. What personal thoughts and feelings arise when you think of red, yellow, green, blue, black, white, and so on?

Also think about where these colours appear in waking life. For example, blue is the colour of the sky and the sea, green is the colour of nature, and so on. And don't forget the use of colour in language: 'seeing red', 'feeling blue', and so on. As with all dream associations, trust your gut reactions and look for the associations that make the most sense to you.

Here are some colour associations and trigger words to help you get to your own personal associations. I also urge you to research the spiritual meanings of any colours that appear in your dreams, as you will find it both helpful and healing.

Beige: Neutral, bland, detached, an absence of passion

Black: Mystery, infinite possibility, death of the old, endings, darkest and deepest fears

Blue: Cool, calming, truth, intellect, justice, communication, wisdom, expansiveness; in dreams blue skies are often believed to be a sign of the conscious mind

Brown: Down-to-earth, grounded, self-sufficiency, practicality, the material

Gold: Wealth, prosperity, success, value

Green: Nature, hope, growth, vitality, healing, jealousy, envy

Grey: Ambiguity, lack of vibrancy

Orange: Creativity, generosity, optimism, warmth, sociability

Pink: Unconditional love, compassion, joy, sweetness

Purple: Royalty, spirituality, dignity, respect

Red: Heat, blood, passion, excitement, lust, anger, stop sign, danger, sexuality

Silver: Skill, luck, protective energy, intuition, the moon

White: Innocence, purity, peace, cleanliness, awareness, reawakening

Yellow: Thoughts, intellect, fear, cowardice, creativity, sunshine

COMMUNICATION

Dreams are communication from your unconscious or true inner self to your conscious self. Once you understand your personal symbolism, the messages being sent to you become easier to decode. But if a dream contains any symbols of communication, such as handwriting, letters, phones, messages, e-mails, and so on, the meaning can be easier to decipher.

When trying to understand these messages, first consider whether the message makes a clear reference to your waking life or triggers other personal associations. Then consider the form the communication took, as a phone call suggests something more immediate and informal than an e-mail. If the message was in a code you can't crack, does that suggest lack of understanding in some area of your waking life?

CONFLICT

Conflict, like change, is an inescapable fact of life, but remember that your dreams always comment on or offer brainstorming solutions to what is happening in your waking life, and understanding the nature of conflict in your life can help you cope with it better.

Conflict themes in dreams are easy to spot and include dreams of arguments, immediate threat or danger, being chased or attacked, falling, drowning, fighting, violence, destruction, weapons and warfare.

If you dream about killing a person or animal or see people or animals being killed, this doesn't mean you have violent tendencies. Instead, it points to the death of mindsets or actions. If poison features, this refers to some undercover action you are taking or which is being taken against you. Look for clues in the dream. Who or what is being killed or poisoned? Think like a dream detective. All the clues are there, if you look closely enough.

And if someone kills you in your dream or you are attacked, this suggests someone or something in your waking life is imposing on you against your will. Find out who or what that is and protect your boundaries.

DISASTERS

Your dreaming mind will often employ symbols of natural disaster, such as volcanoes erupting or forest fires, to convey striking and memorable images or messages. You may wake up feeling terrified and/or concerned for your own safety or that of others, and to dream of a natural disaster is always unnerving, but it is important to point out that such dreams are rarely prophetic; it is more likely that they are an expression of unexpressed or hidden fears concerning events that are beyond your control, for example what the future will bring and what other people think of you. Having said that, always be alert to the fact that sometimes your intuition has noticed things in your waking life that could compromise your safety or well-being, so there's no harm in doing safety checks.

On the other hand, dreams of natural disaster can also point to great inner change, and although this change is important, it can make you feel temporarily uncertain of yourself and your direction in life. Your dreaming mind is helping you process all this uncertainty so you can better deal with it in your waking life.

If the dream disaster is man-made – for example, a crash or an attack or choking – this strongly indicates that something in your waking life urgently needs to change to avoid things going wrong. This could be a relationship, a job or a mindset that isn't optimum for you. Your dreaming mind is using this symbol to let you know that this is something over which you do have control, in contrast to natural-disaster dreams, which tend to depict forces outside your control. Having said that, apocalypse or end-of-the-world dreams or nuclear-war dreams indicate there is some kind of personal upheaval going on that is completely changing your life, such as divorce, job loss, the death of a loved one, and so on, that it feels like the end of your world as you know it.

Apocalyptic or end-of-the-world scenarios may also be a response to terrifying events on the world stage that concern you, but more often than not they point to a seismic change in your waking life that has 'rocked your world'. Things will never be the same again. End-of-the-world dreams may be frequent following the death of a loved one.

This kind of dream is helping you process the enormity of what you are experiencing, while at the same time reminding you that with every ending there is always a new beginning. It is encouraging you to take things slowly, trust that there will be a new dawn and pay close attention to your personal survival needs. In your dream the world ends, but you are one of the survivors, and in your waking life you can survive too.

The details of any disaster dream are important. Is the disaster involving you alone or are you in a group? If it is the latter, it could reflect a social or work experience or encounter, rather than a personal one.

If the disaster isn't the end of the world but instead features a sinking ship or plane or car crash, it is a symbol of something significant in your waking life that has now veered off-course. It is also likely to involve not just yourself but other people. It isn't necessarily going to be harmful, but it is dragging you and others down in some way, so changes in your perspective need to be made. Not surprisingly, many brides planning big weddings experience this kind of dream. The message is not to let the event, however important, drag you down and suck the joy out of it.

To recap: dreaming of any kind of disaster, be it man-made or natural, like a volcano or avalanche, is deeply unsettling, but in virtually all cases it is an expression of fears concerning events that you feel are out of your control, despite your best efforts.

On the other hand, disaster dreams also reveal stunning potential for radical inner growth and transformation. Understanding that there is no point stressing over what you can't control and focusing on what you can – your perspective and your reactions – is the overriding lesson here and the only way forward. To quote the serenity (sweet dreams) prayer:

God, grant me the serenity to accept the things I cannot change, the courage to change the things I can, and the wisdom to know the difference.

ELEMENTS

When the elements of Air, Earth, Fire and Water appear in your dream, they represent the state of your psychological well-being, with Air typically symbolizing thought, Earth sensation, Fire intuition and Water feeling.

Air

Air is inventiveness and versatility as well as freedom and objectivity. If you are conscious of Air-related symbols in your dreams, such as balloons, breathing, storms, flying or falling, these are associated with the realm of thoughts and intellect. Focus on the condition of these symbols and how they make you feel in the dream. Do they raise you up or drag you down?

Earth

The Earth element has ancient associations with the human body and being grounded, practical and realistic, and in dreams, symbols of this element, such as grass, mud, trees, etc., can represent things in your life that you may be taking for granted. Pay attention to the quality of these dream symbols and the associations you have with them. Are they harsh and rough or soft and luscious? Are they thriving or wilting? If mud features, this is a powerful symbol of creation, as things grow in mud and soil.

The Earth element can also symbolize things you have buried in your past.

Fire

Fire is a potent symbol of passion, new beginnings, energy and vitality. It can both create and destroy, so be alert to how it is expressed in your dream. Is some passion in your waking life dying or do you need to take action to energize it?

Water

In dreams, Water is a potent symbol of the dreamer's emotional life. It is also a symbol of the spiritual life-force. In many cultures, to be baptized is to be cleansed and healed and to start afresh. Water is also associated with the fluid in the womb.

Dream oceans and seas represent unconscious emotions or urges that are impacting your waking life. Are you floating, swimming or struggling against the tide in your dreams? However Water appears, it is a symbol of your emotional state or the need to reconnect with and understand parts of yourself that are submerged. If you are washing yourself or something in a dream, this points to the cleansing of negative emotions, such as fear and self-doubt.

EVERYDAY ITEMS

Although you may have your share of fantasy dream scenarios, the chances are your dreams will also be littered with everyday objects. Although some believe this is simply the brain's way of processing things, most dream experts believe that dream objects have symbolic value and represent far more than their everyday function suggests.

The way in which an everyday object or item is used in the dream and the situation it is used in will be key to the interpretation. What is the purpose of the object and what does that purpose have to teach you? In other words, everyday things in dreams operate in much the same way as all symbols, with both personal and shared meanings.

However mundane a symbol may appear, for example a traffic light or a microwave, it matters. Nothing is random or trivial in your dream life. Treat all dream symbols with equal reverence, as all of them have something of value to impart. In a dream, like the night poet you are, you can glimpse heaven in a grain of sand and see possibilities in everything.

FAMILY

A vital part of personal growth is becoming independent of childhood patterns. An absence of a secure family and/or parental love can be deeply traumatic to your sense of self, but even if you came from a happy family, your dreaming mind will still use family members to help you face unresolved conflicts on your path to self-reliance and maturity.

Family-themed dreams are common, because many of our inner conflicts are experienced first within the family. It is as if a pattern has been imprinted and that pattern will continue to repeat until broken willingly.

The way you were raised has a profound effect on your psychological well-being and any dream you have of your parent figure(s) or other family members will be deeply meaningful. So, if a family member appears in a dream, your first task is to define and understand the health of your present relationship with that family member. And as these are people you share your life with on a daily basis, please consider the rare but possible literal interpretation. Is this dream actually about what is going on for them?

Then cast your net wider and consider how family members can represent archetypes or aspects of yourself that you need to nurture for your personal growth. For example, the father traditionally represents assertiveness and authority, the mother protection. If you dream of siblings, this could represent your *anima* and *animus*, the feminine and masculine aspects of your personality, struggling for recognition.

FEAR

Fear and anxiety are the most commonly expressed emotions in dreams, followed closely by anger. To help you identify what is triggering these negative dream feelings, brainstorm your personal associations with the specific dream symbols that inspired them. The answer will be hidden there.

Be aware that your dream is using these symbols to express tension and conflict between your conscious and unconscious –

in other words, your external versus your inner life. The key to finding happiness is to balance these two aspects of yourself, allow them to co-exist in harmony. Dream work is a perfect way to find that balance.

If you are overcome with feelings of panic, horror and fear in a dream, this classifies as a nightmare. Terrifying and hostile dreams draw your attention shockingly and sharply to the many hidden fears that may be preventing you from moving forward in your waking life. They are seminal dreams and the advice coming up in the next lesson will help you understand that, like all dreams, nightmares are priceless transformative gifts, once you know how to process them.

FINDING
Finding a secret room

If you discover a secret room that has been long forgotten, this clearly suggests a neglected part of your life that your dreaming mind is encouraging you to reclaim. It is telling you it isn't too late to learn a skill, travel, follow your heart, and so on.

If what you find in the room is frightening, this reflects insights you find hard to face in your waking life but need to deal with for your personal growth.

If there are windows in the secret room, this may offer a clue to the meaning, as windows offer a view or perspective of the outside world and signify your outlook on life. Eyes are sometimes called windows to the soul. Is the view clear or are the windows shut, suggesting a shuttered outlook on life? Is it time to let in some fresh air and daylight?

Finding valuables

Finding hidden treasure or cash or winning the lottery points to the discovery of something precious within you.

FISH

In Jungian dream analysis, fish and underwater dreams represent the deepest levels of your unconscious mind, so their appearance could point to deep-rooted fears that haven't surfaced in waking life. They could also symbolize the spiritual journey, though, as well as abundance. Given all these possible interpretations, it is important to consider your personal associations with these objects and the condition and appearance of the fish.

If a whale appears in your dreams, this is often a potent symbol of power and hope, reassurance that a huge healing and spiritually transformative force within you is awakening.

And, as with all dream interpretations, consider whether your unconscious is using word play, puns or idioms to get its point across. For example, 'fish out of water', 'fishing for something', 'whale of a time', and so on.

FLOWERS

The fragile beauty of a flower has long been regarded as a symbol of the spiritual self and pure inner beauty.

If flowers appear in your dream, pay attention to their type and both the personal and common symbolism there. For starters, roses are associated with romantic love, daisies with innocence, and so on. Then note the symbolism of the colour of the flowers as well as their condition. Are they fresh or wilting?

In general, though flowers may well point to the cycle of birth and death – not surprisingly, they often appear in dreams of departed loved ones – they also symbolize your inner beauty bursting through. Tend your dream flowers.

FOOD AND DRINK

Dreams about food and drink may reference actual hunger and thirst, but more often than not, these are symbols for other appetites, for example for spiritual, emotional, sexual and intellectual nourishment.

According to Jung, dream food suggests the qualities you are taking in or need to take in for your personal, emotional and spiritual development. In other words, the dream is trying to compensate for malnourishment in some area of your life. Your task is to identify what that area of deficiency is.

Dreams about eating, drinking, cooking, dining, fasting or gorging point to your current state of psychological well-being.

And if a specific food or drink is highlighted in your dream, this is significant, as different foods and drinks can mean different things and have different associations. For instance, bread typically represents what sustains you, the basics of life, and so on. Go directly for your personal associations before researching common or universal associations with the food and drink of your dreams.

FOREIGN COUNTRIES

Should you find yourself visiting, holidaying, observing or living in a foreign country in your dreams, this is all about your attitude to opinions that are different from your own. It can also be about meeting an aspect of yourself that feels unfamiliar.

Your associations, beliefs and opinions about your dream country need to be investigated first. Do any aspects of your waking life connect with what you glimpsed in your dream?

While hearing a foreign or strange language in a dream can be a symbol of misunderstandings, it can also point to some kind of communication block within you, something important that has not yet become clear enough for you to understand or put into words.

If the country you find yourself in is totally unfamiliar or unheard of, this can point to how well you are coping with a significant change.

Whether you are familiar with the foreign country or not, pay attention to all the details and how the people react to you there, as they all provide clues to the interpretation.

GATHERINGS

Groups or gatherings, such as weddings, crowds or parties, in a dream are all about how you relate to others in your waking life. If you find yourself in a dream gathering, the best way to start interpreting this dream is to consider the reason for the gathering, the atmosphere there and the feeling generated within you. These will spotlight your perceived status within your family, social and professional life, and any insecurities you may have.

Dream groups can represent both your strengths and your anxieties when it comes to relating to and mixing with others. As social relationships are vital for your psychological well-being, dream gatherings can help clarify your way of interacting with others and what is working and what isn't. Pay attention to how the people in your dream gatherings react to you, as that can help you understand better how you are being perceived by others.

GIFTS

Giving and receiving gifts in dreams indicates a need to balance give and take within a relationship as well as a need to recognize your own worth.

Receiving an unwanted gift in a dream could suggest unwelcome attention from someone in your waking life or intrusive negative thoughts. An empty gift box warns against taking things at face value.

HOLIDAYS

If your dreaming mind takes you on holiday, much will depend on how you feel. If you have packed too many bags or are struggling to carry them, you have emotional baggage you need to leave behind. However, if you are sunning yourself on an idyllic beach with gentle waves lapping against the shore, this could be your dreaming mind treating you to a mini holiday to motivate you. This could also suggest a longing to escape your daily routine. You, and only you, can decide.

HOME

You may find that your dreaming mind often places you in your home or a place you have once lived. Dream homes say very little about your real-life residence and a great deal about you.

According to Jung, all the developmental stages of your life and parts of your conscious and unconscious self are represented by dream homes. So, when trying to analyse your dream home, consider how it is kept and its condition, colour and shape, and the different rooms, as they all relate to aspects of your personality. When a dream shows you in a particular home, your dreaming mind is letting you now this is where you are coming from right now and this is how things are affecting you. If you find yourself in your childhood home, what lessons from the past can you apply to the present?

Dream homes also suggest returning to yourself or finding a space where you can breathe easy and be yourself without fear of reprisal. Spiritualists speak of 'going home' when they talk about the afterlife, as they believe the physical state is a temporary one.

One of the most commonly reported dream home scenarios is being in your home or a place you are familiar with and you suddenly discover a room or cupboard or place you didn't know was there before, which suggests a neglected part of your life that your dreaming mind is encouraging you to reclaim. It is telling you it isn't too late to learn a skill, travel, follow your heart, and so on. (*See also Finding.*)

And if you dream of a burglar trying to break into your house, first of all make sure your home is safe in waking life. Then consider the symbolism of an intruder. It indicates an unwelcome and uninvited presence in your life. Consider whether unusual things are happening in your waking life. Has someone or something invaded your personal or emotional space, perhaps a new workplace or a new group of friends?

A change is as good as a rest, and in waking life you may quite rightly be trying to make the best of upheavals, but your dreaming mind is suggesting you do a risk assessment and urging you to not let your guard down until safe to do so. This nocturnal forewarning can help you take off the rose-tinted glasses and see things in your life as the complicated kaleidoscope of colours and shades that they are.

INSECTS

Insects are irritating and potentially dangerous creatures that can attack without warning in great numbers, causing illness and in some cases death. So, if they appear in your dreams, what (or who) is infesting your life?

Although insect-related dreams are generally warning you about a small irritation in your waking life, it is important to point out that insects often have qualities we admire. For example, ants are hard-working, bees make honey, spiders are ingenious, and so on. Use your common sense and some general associations when interpreting dreams that feature insects.

And in your research don't neglect the importance of learning about your dream insect, because nature is a great teacher. Perhaps something in how that creature survives can offer you commentary or advice on how to cope better in your waking life?

(See also Spiders.)

JEWELLERY

Jewellery in dreams suggests something precious of unique personal value to you. This also applies to crystals, gemstones and rocks in a dream. Pay attention to the condition of the gem, its colour and any symbolic associations, such as whether it is a birthstone or not, as that could be spotlighting characteristics associated with that month or zodiac sign. As with every dream symbol, start with the personal, and if nothing resonates, cast your net wide when you brainstorm for associations and wait until one clearly resonates, because that means you have struck decoding gold.

JOY

Should you wake up with feelings of joy without knowing why, chances are your dreaming mind has given you an emotional boost in a dream filled with happy and loving symbols.

Such dreams are less common than anxiety-related ones because life is a series of challenges and your dreams are always trying to problem-solve what is happening in your reality. However, joyous dreams are just as important to decode as negative ones, because they offer you an opportunity to reflect on the experiences and situations that evoked them and how you can recreate that feeling in your waking life.

To encourage more joy-filled dreams, try some daydreaming during waking hours. Watch videos of birds flying in your mind just before you fall asleep. Imagine how it feels to see the world from their perspective. You can also imagine setting sail on a great adventure. And if you do recall amazing dreams on waking, be sure to write them down. Celebrate your happy dreams as much as you can.

Although positive experiences are usually less common in dreams than negative ones, when they do appear, their purpose is to compensate and motivate. Be aware that sometimes your dreaming mind will send you a dream to compensate for negative experiences in your waking life. For example, if you feel unhappy, you may wake up having dreamed of winning the lottery or being awarded a Nobel Prize. The purpose of such dreams is to help you believe in yourself and draw on your inner courage. Your dreaming mind is giving you a vote of confidence. This is the case, too, if you find yourself being the superhero in your dreams. The message is that if you follow and believe in your dreams, you can find ways to overcome roadblocks in your waking life.

Hopefully, by the time you finish reading this book and complete all the exercises, including the vital ones in the final lesson, which encourage you to incubate healing dreams, you will find that more and more of your dreams feature good deeds, promising signs and happy things. If you can dream of these things, this means your unconscious believes you are capable of them, and what you unconsciously believe you are capable of is often what you attract or manifest in your waking life.

Good dreams, good life.

LEISURE ACTIVITIES

If one of your favourite leisure activities features in your dreams, chances are your dreaming mind is urging you to take some time out of a busy schedule to do the things you love to do. It could also suggest ways in which you can improve your current experience or become more accomplished by transferring some of the skills from the leisure activity to a current waking challenge. This is especially the case if the leisure activity is something you wouldn't dream of doing in your waking life, for example hang-gliding.

Take note also whether the leisure activity is a solo or a group one, as your dreaming mind may be urging you to be more reflective and self-reliant or to reach out for the advice and support of others.

Should gambling be a dream theme, this suggests that you feel as if your destiny is not in your own hands and your dreaming mind may be urging you to only take risks that are calculated.

If chess appears in your dream, this represents the need for some strategy in your waking life to help you overcome the odds. It can also point to black and white thinking.

Dreaming of watching a movie or play in a theatre could suggest that you may need to distance yourself from some drama in your waking life or, depending on your personal associations, stop passively watching and get more involved in the action.

Should childhood toys appear in your dreams, take note. This could be a reminder to introduce more fun into your waking life. It could also be urging you to put your energy to more productive use. Again, your intuition will tell you which interpretation is correct for you.

LETTERS OF THE ALPHABET

If your dreaming mind draws your attention to a specific letter, brainstorm all possible personal and common associations with that letter. For example, the letter 'A' suggests excellence, a note on the musical scale, a vitamin or any place, name or word beginning with that letter. Keep brainstorming until you get that moment of clarity.

LOSS AND FRUSTRATION

Dreams that have themes of loss include losing teeth and hair, getting lost or losing loved ones, a body part or even your own life.

In some instances, these loss dreams are your dreaming mind helping you process actual events or people you have lost, but in most cases they will symbolize something missing in your life, perhaps direction, confidence or intimacy, or even a sense of personal identity.

Loss dreams could also be a warning that you are in danger of losing something or someone that matters to you, or that you aren't valuing an aspect of your life enough. They could also be metaphors for lost opportunities or forgotten aspects of yourself.

As always, your personal associations with the thing(s) you lose in the dream will give you clues to the interpretation.

Frustration-themed dreams are similar and include dreams about being paralysed, imprisoned, chased, falling, failing an examination, forgetting lines, missing a train or plane, running late, being inappropriately dressed and struggling with malfunctioning technology.

Try to pinpoint the cause of any feelings of loss and frustration in the dream, because identifying that cause will help identify that factor in your waking life.

However upsetting or painful these dreams may be, they aren't meant to cause you anxiety. Your dreaming mind has conjured up these symbols to inform and strengthen you, so that if faced with loss and frustration in your waking life, you have been there before, felt the fear and know you can conquer it.

LOVE

If love is a key theme in your dream – if you fall in love or feel great love, or encounter symbols of love such as a dove, a heart or shooting an arrow – this dream may be urging you to inject more love into your own life, starting with loving yourself.

MAGIC

You could say that every dream has its own magic, but if any mystical arts emerge as symbols in your dream, such as astrology, the Tarot, spells, shamans, crystals, and so on, the first thing is to consider your attitude towards the mystical arts in waking life. Do you regard anything magical as fraudulent or do you believe there is something in it? Your attitude will influence your interpretation of the dream.

Whether you believe there are magical elements in your life or not, your first introduction to the mystical would likely have been in your childhood, with fairy tales, and vestiges of those fairy tales and the archetypal images found in them will linger in your unconscious and resurface in your dreams. For example, if you meet someone that you instinctively dislike, your feelings towards them may be symbolized in a dream by the appearance of a witch or evil sorcerer.

Whatever you feel about the mystical arts, should your dreaming mind settle on an image related to one of them, for example a Tarot card, you have everything to gain and nothing to lose by bringing your dream to life and doing your own research into that card. None of the mystical arts have any sinister or evil powers. The power is always in you and what you choose to believe.

Bear in mind that your dream work might be considerably enhanced and deepened by researching and working with the archetypal images of astrology and the Tarot. Indeed, Jung saw all Tarot cards as being 'descended from the archetypes of transformation'.

MEDIA AND TECHNOLOGY

Although we live in a time when phones, social media and technology appear to dominate our lives, interestingly, dreaming about mobiles and computers isn't as common as you would think. This is because the dreaming mind in its infinite wisdom knows that true meaning can't be found in technology.

Should computers, TVs, phones and technology feature in your dream, they could be reflections of your day-to-day preoccupation with them, but are far more likely to symbolize the rational, unemotional part of your mind or your stored memories. Internet-themed dreams point to limitless possibilities as well as connections.

Phones are typically a symbol of communication or a desire to make contact with an aspect of yourself or someone else you need to say something important to. An unanswered dream phone suggests ignoring something or someone by refusing to see or hear it/them. If you pick up your dream phone, then there is information available to you that you do not consciously know.

Televisions can represent your thoughts, and radio your inner voice. Notice what is on the TV or radio in your dream and remember that the purpose of TV and radio is to entertain, inform and distract. Your dreaming mind may be using a scene from a TV show to symbolize a current concern to you.

Social media themes appearing in dreams often relate to the image you want to present to the world and the way you interact with or reach out to others. For example, losing followers suggests feeling neglected or distant from others, and so on.

Focus on how the media in your dream makes you feel or what insights it triggers.

MONEY

Money in dreams represents things of value to you, but not necessarily monetary value. However, if cash, coins, jewels, treasure or a lottery win appear in your dreams, first try to identify what money means to you in a non-materialistic sense. This dream theme is trying to help you become aware of what you truly value in life as well as what price you are prepared to pay for your actions and desires.

Think symbolically. It may be that gold doesn't represent the precious metal to you, but someone with a heart of gold, just as a dream of treasure may represent people in your life that you treasure.

What are your associations with money? Do you associate it with freedom, power, attractiveness and self-confidence? Pondering such questions may help you identify what is of true value and what the real price of your previous goals and ambitions has been.

NATURE

Dreams that feature natural images and settings may be related to those parts of your being that are natural or not moulded by conscious ambitions and desires. In ancient religions, nature was thought to be alive with a multitude of spirits and your dreaming mind may use images of nature to help you meet primordial aspects of your unconscious.

Nature in dreams can also represent the nurturing mother archetype and the sense of being grounded or connected to the Earth. It may therefore represent your essence, unaffected by personality traits, or something that feels natural or second nature to you. Remember too that the great outdoors is often said to be relaxing and calming, and your dreaming mind may be prompting you to take some time out from your busy routine.

Be aware that natural symbols will be rich in associations, both personal and common. For example, a forest has sexual associations as well as personal growth and spiritual ones. A field suggests freedom and happiness, a mountain a challenge to climb, plants are a wise life-force, and rivers, seas, oceans and lakes serve as a reminder that change and renewal can be refreshing rather than fearful experiences. Trees are archetypal symbols of the process of growth and reaching for enlightenment.

The interpretation of these symbols, as with all your dreams, will be a combination of your own personal associations and universal ones, and much will also depend on their condition in your dream. Is the grass in the field lush and green, suggesting new hope, or is it downtrodden and parched, suggesting the importance of refreshment and basic self-care?

Take note of any seasonal references in your dreams too. Autumn tends to be associated with maturity and the beauty of letting go; winter with later years of your life and contemplation; spring with youth, optimism and rebirth; and summer with relaxation and fulfilment.

NUMBERS

When a number appears in your dreams, first take note of any personal associations with that number, as it may have relevance to your waking world. For example, the number of your children, your age or days of the week, or years, or phone numbers, and so on. Your mind may often retain the significance of a number or date even if you don't consciously recall it. So do some research.

If you can't figure out any personal associations, the next step is to go for the symbolic meanings of the number or numbers. If you see a series of numbers, add them together so they make one digit and then research the symbolism of that number. Numbers have had symbolic significance within all cultures, religions and belief systems in the world. In numerology, they point to both inner and outer spiritual forces.

Dream numbers may also reference time running out or the importance of making a calculated move. Odd numbers are considered to be more passive and even numbers more active.

Numerology is an absolutely fascinating field of study and researching it for yourself will complement your dream work, as numbers do represent archetypal energies and the various stages of personal and spiritual growth. For a snapshot: one is typically a symbol of intention and independence; two of the drive towards companionship; three of creativity; four of building foundations; five of transformation; six of family and relationships; seven of intuition; eight of material success; and nine of wisdom and completion.

PEOPLE

Chances are, whatever age and stage of life you are in, you will repeatedly dream of other people at some point. Sometimes these will be loved ones and family members, or perhaps they will be old friends, colleagues or people you haven't been in touch with for years, or even total strangers.

Given that facial recognition in dreams and in waking life activates the same part of the brain, the people in your dreams will often feel incredibly realistic.

You may think that when you see another person in your dreams, the dream is about that person. This is rarely the case.

When people appear in your dreams, it is typically because they are associated with certain personality traits that you need to understand better. The dream should be interpreted subjectively, so whenever you encounter another person in your dreams, ask yourself, 'What is the single word that describes that person?' Then ask yourself, 'What is the person doing in the dream that I am doing or feeling in my waking life?' Consider, too, if you admire or envy that person.

People in your dreams can raise issues you would rather forget. But if you listen to your dream characters, they may be able to help you deal with current waking challenges and find inner balance.

Always consider the feelings the dream inspires in you, the role the character played in it and your waking association with them. What is all this saying about you?

At times you may dream of archetypes or people you don't know but who appear like a one-dimensional, stereotypical character in a 'B' movie, for example a detective or a soldier or a nun or a servant. In the dream you know what their role is, but you have never met them in real life. Generic characters like this represent aspects of yourself that you need to understand and give a better script or presence to in your waking life.

Having said that, if the dream characters resemble famous fictional characters, you may want to consider if they are representing aspects of someone you have feelings for or an emotional reaction to. The joy of reading fiction comes from the empathy we develop for the characters, so perhaps your dreaming mind is urging you to have greater empathy for someone in your life who displays aspects of that fictional character.

The people you are closest to – your partner, children, family and loved ones – don't typically represent aspects of you in a dream and are more likely to point to your relationship with the real person. Your dreaming mind is trying to help you understand their perspective better so your relationship can improve. How the person you are close to appears in the dream will be key to your interpretation.

Often your dreaming mind will recognize a repeating relationship pattern in your waking life and use characters from your past to highlight that pattern to you. On other occasions, repeating characters from your past will indicate qualities within yourself that you are denying, have forgotten or need to understand better.

In general, if you dream of someone from your past and the relationship was a painful one, this suggests those painful patterns are repeating and the lesson needs to be relearned in the present. However, if you dream of people from your past who were supportive of you, this is a sign that with a dose of self-belief anything is possible for you.

If the recurring character is a celebrity or famous person, in much the same way as generic dream characters, focus on what qualities you most associate with them and how you can ignite that essence or energy within yourself. Your dreaming mind is suggesting that developing those qualities may help you navigate your current challenges.

On the other hand, a famous person can also represent your hidden side or shadow, or a part of your personality or a behaviour pattern that you have hidden or feel unable to face. Often this happens in childhood, when our parents or carers praise certain behaviours and disapprove of others, so we learn to bury behaviours that are disapproved of because our survival depends on our parents' protection and approval. Sometimes these hidden aspects of ourselves can be negative traits, such as jealousy and spite, but they can be positive ones too. For example, if as a child you were taught to be seen and not heard, the assertive aspects of your personality will be hidden in your shadow. Shining a light on your shadow will not only help you understand yourself better, but can also release hidden potential that you should connect to.

Of course, if you dream of a stranger, then this almost certainly represents the parts of yourself that you are unaware of, your shadow. When you gain insight into what qualities within yourself your dream character is highlighting, the meaning of your dream will materialize.

PRIZES

Dreams of being suddenly famous or receiving trophies, prizes and awards usually reflect a need to be recognized and respected by others, but could also be your dreaming mind urging greater self-belief.

PROBLEMS

Dreams are the small hidden door to the deepest and most mysterious part of yourself. They act as teachers and guides down the royal road towards psychological healing. In essence, your dreams all present to you, in symbolic language, the challenges you are facing in waking life, so you can understand them and yourself better. These challenges can often be represented by symbols that you can make personal associations with or easily find common associations with, but sometimes those symbols are puzzles that appear to defy all explanation.

Dreams that fall into this category are dreams in which you find yourself presented with some insurmountable problem or difficulty – wading through a bog, fighting rain and snow, struggling to climb over a fence, being lost in a maze, failing to untie a knot or unlock a door or solve a mystery, and so on. It may simply be that you have, without realizing it, lost your sense of direction in your waking life, so to help you flex and tone your problem-solving skills, your dreaming mind is presenting you with a challenge.

Life is a great mystery and it is impossible to understand everything about it and about your inner world. Since dreams reflect life, it isn't surprising that some of them are as mysterious and unsolvable as life itself.

If you do have a dream that defies explanation, keep reflecting on it and ask your dreaming mind to send you another dream that makes things clearer.

If you believe the dream is about a situation in your waking life but can't understand the message, reflect on that waking situation before you go to sleep to give your dreaming mind a directive. State your request to recall and understand your dreams clearly and directly to your dreaming mind before you go to sleep. Sometimes you may have to do this over several nights, depending on how in harmony your conscious and unconscious minds are.

Just as it can help to think of problems as puzzles, sometimes when things seem to be falling apart in your dreams and in your waking life, perhaps they are falling into place.

Your Life in your Dreams

Inexplicable dreams can help you cathartically process unanswered questions about those times when there seems to be no justice in the world.

Perhaps this metaphor will help: dreams that are impossible to understand are like attempts to make sense of the messy knots and loose ends on the underside of a tapestry. Sometimes the connections will make some sense, but it is only when you turn the tapestry over and get to see the bigger picture – often by recording your dreams over a lengthy period of time – that they can make real sense.

RELIGION

Should religious symbols or themes appear in your dreams, it is essential to take your own beliefs into consideration. If you are religious, the dream may simply be urging you to make decisions in line with your faith. But if you dream of a belief system that is not yours, your dreaming mind may be urging you to inject a hefty dose of sacred respect for your inner space into your life.

SCHOOL

All dreams are your teachers and guides in the school of self-healing, so dreams that feature schools and teachers are especially significant.

If a dream takes you back to school, it will be focusing on lessons you learned or failed to learn then, and these lessons may be relevant to or repeating in your waking life. For example, in the dream you may be unprepared for an exam or have lost your homework or text books or be struggling to get your locker or desk open, even though everyone around you is coping fine. These dreams are often accompanied by feelings of both frustration and embarrassment. In this case, your dreaming mind is trying to tell you that there may be things in your school locker that represent authentic parts of yourself, or even the real you, that you feel cut off from.

Many people who have these 'back to school' and feeling cut-off dreams aren't typically struggling socially, but still have something vibrant, creative and authentic within them that they need to reconnect with.

This dream is also urging you to stop trying so hard to fit in and to focus your energy on self-understanding instead.

SENSES

Sometimes you may recall a dream where you heard birds singing or saw a sunset or smelled perfume or touched a flame or tasted champagne. If this is the case, your dreaming mind is doubling down and offering you intense realism to urge waking action or a change of perspective. And sometimes intensely vivid dreams can take you into lucid dreaming territory (see page 244).

Focus on which of the senses was most realistic in your dream – hearing, sight, taste, touch, smell – and in your waking life, notice that sense or senses as never before to see what you can learn. Also consider all the personal and common associations with those senses and what they might convey to you. For instance, if touching things was vivid in your dream, do you need to reach out to someone or something or do you need to get in touch with your own feelings?

And should your dreams feature sixth-sense themes, such as telepathy or precognition, refer to page 224.

SETTING, LOCATION

The setting or location of a dream suggests how a situation in your waking life is impacting you emotionally. It is often a vivid clue about the dream topic, and commonly a metaphor. For example, a sunny scene could be optimism, or the need for it, and a grey landscape a gloomy view.

As fascinating as the other symbols in your dream may be, they only really make sense when interpreted within the setting of the dream. For example, a dream prison setting suggests feeling trapped, a thunderstorm suggests heartbreak, and so on. The aim is to help you acknowledge the role of your emotions and how they are derailing you, so that you can gift yourself a much-needed dose of self-awareness and accompanying compassion.

Try to assign a feeling and a function to the specific setting of your dream. For example, a busy city setting suggests the feeling of purpose and speed. Then see how the feeling and function comment on your own inner landscape. Bear in mind that the weather, the lighting, the structure and other features of your dreamscape contribute to the setting and are all saying something about your mood or state of mind. This is especially the case if your dream features extremes of temperature or if the weather is uncharacteristic in some ways, such as snow falling in summer.

It is also worthwhile contemplating your position within the dream, as this can give you an indication of your stance towards something in your waking life or how you are currently handling a situation. If you are in a raised position, this suggests a wider perspective is needed. If you are adjacent to or beside someone or something, this suggests a close connection or something you can no longer avoid. If you are looking down, this points to the need for greater optimism to raise you up.

SEX AND EROTICA

Things can frequently get both intense and steamy in dreamland and you may find yourself waking up feeling deeply involved and touched. Your dreaming mind is using the metaphor of sex to help you better understand not just your relationships but yourself.

To help you find this understanding, your dreaming mind will throw all your relationship history – both positive and negative – at you, as well as all the associations you have with romance and love. It does this to help you experiment with situations and emotions you may not allow yourself to experience in your waking life for fear of hurting or betraying those closest to you.

It seems that throughout your life your dreaming mind never stops reflecting on your intimate relationships and what you can learn from them. It is always trying to make sense of what went wrong and conjuring up what can work out better next time. However, the way it does this shifts according to your age and life stage.

In your teens, dreams often present erotic scenarios with people you know in your waking life, leaving you waking up wondering if you really fancy them or they fancy you. Sometimes that is the case, but more often than not it is your dreaming mind cathartically exploring your preoccupation with sex.

In your twenties and thirties, dream lovers tend to be people you don't know or whom you aren't attracted to at all in waking life. These dreams are usually about assimilating the qualities of the person rather than the person themself.

Your thirties and forties are also the decades in which dreams of an ex may rise to the surface. This is because your dreaming mind is encouraging you to reflect on how your old relationship broke down so you can make different decisions in the future. Rest assured your dreaming mind isn't urging you to reach out to your ex; it's simply using them as a symbol to comment on your current relationship. It is also doing what it does your entire life, which is to help you learn from past experiences so you can heal your present and look forward to a better future. It is sorting through what worked and what didn't work, rather like a nocturnal filing system dedicated to your complicated heart. Every dream is trying to ensure that moving forward, you can love more deeply and more successfully.

In later life, sexual dreams may reference lovers or people from your past to clearly depict specific qualities about them and how they have contributed to your current understanding of love. It seems as if the dreaming mind really wants to zero in on matters of the heart and better understanding the meaning of love, independent of physical desire.

Whatever age you are, if you have a sexual dream about someone who isn't your partner, don't take this as a sign you are about to cheat. It is simply your curious mind offering you a way to adventure and experience safely in a way that can harm absolutely no one. And whether you are in a relationship or not, your dream lover represents *qualities* within yourself and others that you want to sample.

Bear in mind that your dreaming mind loves to be contrary, and dreams featuring symbols not related to sex or erotica are more likely to have a sexual interpretation than dreams which depict literal sex. For example, snakes in dreams can have sexual associations. However, if your dream strongly features sexual themes, first of all consider whether it is a metaphor for genuine sexual feelings you may have towards someone. If that is not the case – and chances are it won't be – then as with cheating dreams (*see page 85*), explore what the metaphor of sex suggests to you.

Sex is about getting aroused and the coming together of two separate parties. It is also about how much energy or vibes you have tied up in a specific relationship or area of your life, or how much libido – or life-force – is pulsating through you.

The Freudian interpretation that all dreams are sexual wish-fulfilment lingers. But we most certainly don't always dream about sex and not all dream symbols have an erotic interpretation. Sex is a universal symbol for fertility, the creative life-force and the union of opposites, the masculine and feminine traits within you, so these are all meanings you can consider.

The emotional tone of the dream will suggest what in your waking life is turning you on or off. If you feel ashamed or the sex is bad, this suggests you are allowing insecurities to repress your natural instincts or urges. If you are enjoying your dream sex, this suggests that in your waking life, pouring yourself into what excites you is the only way forward.

Given the central importance of sex, love and relationships in our lives, you may not be surprised to hear that these are the dreams I get by far the most queries about. Most people want to know if a dream lover is interested in them in real life, and the answer is probably not, unless they have shown interest in them in waking life. Dream lovers are most often aspects of yourself you need to foster greater intimacy with. If the dream lover is someone you find unattractive, there may be an unconscious attraction or you could be connecting to them mentally or in a different way than the physical. It's far more likely, though, that the dream is pointing to aspects of yourself that need attention.

If you dream you are the opposite sex, your dreaming mind wants you to explore a different perspective, one typically associated with that gender. For example, if you are a man dreaming you are a woman, this may be urging greater empathy, and if you are a woman dreaming you are a man, this may be spotlighting a need for greater assertiveness.

Incest dreams are deeply unsettling, but they are rarely wish-fulfilment or buried memories. Instead, they suggest that either something in your personal life feels unwholesome in some way or that someone you are currently involved with is getting too close and there is a crossing of boundaries.

If your love-making is interrupted or you can't find anywhere to make love in your dream, this is a representation of outside forces placing barriers into your life that prevent true intimacy. Remember that intimacy may not involve another person, but can also be getting to know yourself better.

Should your relationship be on display to others in the dream, you may be feeling that the judgement or expectations of others regarding your relationship are jeopardizing it.

Dreams of a lover vanishing suggest that you need to see and hold on to what you need in order to feel connected to yourself and others.

Dreaming of making love to a faceless stranger is a call to let go of limiting thoughts, beliefs and ideas and to acknowledge you deserve to experience pleasure.

Sex dreams are the ones that you may find it hardest of all to talk about with other people or to ask advice on because of the potential for embarrassment. Hopefully, the above has reassured you that they are completely natural and entirely positive opportunities to learn more about yourself. However, if you still feel unsettled by them, when you go about the business of decoding them, sticking to the following guidelines will keep you on the straight and narrow:

- *Don't feel guilty.* You understand now that like a great poet or artist, your dreams will use sexual imagery to convey a message. Don't fear them. Understand them instead, because when you do, the guilt will melt away.

- *Focus on the lesson.* What is the dream teaching you about your experience of love? Is it helping you consider someone else's viewpoint? Is it encouraging you to experiment and role-play (safely)?

Your Life in your Dreams

Keep it to yourself. I'm a powerful advocate of dream sharing, with the exception of erotic dreams. These are between you and your dream journal alone and best not shared with loved ones, friends or colleagues.

Appreciate the healing. Remind yourself that however bizarre or corrupt an erotic dream may feel when you recall it on waking, there is always an empowering lesson or deep healing intention behind it.

SHAPES

It is common for shapes and patterns to be a factor in dreams, so don't neglect them when you write in your dream journal. For example, if there was a book in your dream and it was shaped like a triangle, you need to reflect on the symbolism of both book and triangle.

Shapes and patterns in dreams are visual representations of your inner world. For example, circles are typically expressions of infinity, but they also contain and restrict. Triangles represent the trinity and the power of three. Squares are stable and well ordered. Stars are symbols of aspiration and success, and so on.

SHOPPING

Shopping and buying themes in dreams indicate what you think you need to acquire or assimilate in your waking life for your personal happiness. These themes can also point to attitudes you can choose from, decisions you can make or opportunities you are searching for. The key word here is *choice*, as your dreaming mind uses shopping symbols to remind you that you have the power to choose your thoughts and actions.

SICKNESS

Unless you are actually ill, dreams in which your physical health is highlighted typically comment on your emotional and psychological condition. They can represent areas of potential conflict.

If any area of your body is highlighted in a dream, there is no harm making sure you are well, as illness has been diagnosed from a dream before. However, in the great majority of cases, your dreaming mind is using areas of your body as symbols for other areas of your life. Your role is to make a link between your dream ailment and your waking life. Part of your inner world isn't as healthy as it should be.

If blood features in your dreams, consider all the associations. For example, blood is a symbol of life itself, and if you are losing blood, you may be losing moral or physical strength in your waking life. Bones represent structure and support, and so on.

The interpretation of any dream deformity or loss of limbs will depend on which body part is lost or disfigured and the associations you make with that body part. Your dreaming mind will be spotlighting something in your life that you find distasteful. Work out what it is.

And should hospitals, medicine or doctors figure, you are being urged to take control of a situation in your waking life, rather than rely on others.

SPACE

Outer space represents the ultimate in mystery, challenge and unexplored potential in dreams, as in waking life. If any universe/space-related themes, such as the sun, moon, the stars and planets, emerge in your dreams, check in with your personal associations and then enjoy researching common associations. Seek out new horizons. You will find infinite ones. Reflect on them all until something resonates with you and your current circumstances.

SPEECH

If you find yourself talking or hearing a language you don't understand, does this suggest you are missing the point in some area of your life?

SPIRITS AND AFTERLIFE DREAMS

See Lesson 4, page 203.

SURREALISM

Dreaming is surreal. Period. But sometimes your dreaming mind will conjure up super-fantastical images, such as unicorns, fairies and dragons, and when it does, it is a sign you are being powerfully influenced by unconscious forces.

In dreams, fantasy is unlimited and moral judgement suspended, along with logic and reason. Dreams are therefore a way to reveal your deepest desires, and the fantasies you experience there can speak volumes about you, often helping you tackle problems you might normally repress or deny.

If you can understand what a dream is highlighting, you can gain important insight into yourself. Dreams featuring magical, mythical, fairy-tale or fictional beings, things and settings, have one purpose and one purpose alone – they want to help you identify an out-of-the-box approach you may not have considered before, but might want to.

TIME

Dreams exist outside linear time, so if they highlight watches, clocks, calendars, day and night, light and darkness, photographs, time travel or any other literal or symbolic markers of physical time, be sure to take note. Your dreaming mind is telling you loud and clear that right now time is precious and you need to make the most of every moment. It could also be warning you not to be ruled by the clock, or endless to dos in your waking life.

If you time travel to the past in your dreams, research that era and its themes and how they might apply to your waking life. For instance, the Victorian era was known for high morals masking hypocrisy, and so on.

And should you travel to the future, notice every single detail. Your dreaming mind in its infinite mystery may be giving you a sneak preview of what is to come, or reminding you that there is a visionary within you.

TRAVEL AND MOTION

Just as dream cars, planes, bikes and other vehicles are all symbols of the direction your life is heading in, as a rule of thumb any movement or motion in a dream – be that walking, running, flying, dancing – is a commentary on your current progress in waking life and your travels through your inner world.

Travel dreams can be helpful, as they show you what is keeping you from getting where you want to go in life.

Be aware of your dream mode of transport – car, bike, plane, train, etc. – or sense of motion – walking, running, swimming, etc. – along with your emotional reaction to it, as this will all give you a sense of the progress you are making in waking life. Brainstorm the personal and then the common symbolism of the mode of transport as well as the motion. Are you in the driver's seat, and if not, why not?

Should you miss a bus, plane or taxi in a dream, look closely at what you could have done differently to make that connection.

If you take the wrong mode of transport in a dream, this is spotlighting your decision-making process. Is it being influenced by others rather than your own sense of what is right?

And if you are suddenly called to captain or steer the vehicle, this suggests you have been thrust into a position of authority and others are relying on you.

If you are struggling to walk up a steep hill or encountering obstacles that block your momentum in a dream, these all represent personal challenges that make you feel your waking life is a struggle. Your dreaming mind is using this symbolism to help you brainstorm strategies that can help you move forward as well as reminding you that sometimes the only way out is through.

The journey of 1,000 miles begins with one small step, and nothing that is worth achieving happens easily and overnight, so try to think of the obstacles in your path as challenges designed to help you grow stronger and wiser. Overcoming them with patience and hard work will take you one step closer to where you want to be. Slow and steady wins the race.

If you are simply unable to move at all in your dream or are paralysed, this is a sign from your dreaming mind that action must be taken in your waking life to help you move forward. Perhaps you need to leave a job or end a relationship or assert yourself to a loved one, but can't find the courage. If this is the case, the source of the inability to move is within you. You need to shake off an 'I can't do this' mentality, and the best way to do this is to practise self-care, reach out for support from those you trust and take small but steady assertive steps until you can see the way ahead more clearly.

VIOLENCE

Any violence or toxic behaviour in a dream is typically commenting on your own inner conflicts or the hidden parts of yourself you aren't acknowledging. By conjuring up these hidden tensions, your dreaming mind is encouraging you to bring them into the light of day, so they have less hold over you and you reduce the risk of projecting your hidden conflicts onto other people.

Although dreams about violence, crime and other bad actions do reveal your hidden tensions, they can also reveal your feelings about a situation or in some cases your feelings about other people in your life. They are unnerving, and unfortunately more common than positive dream actions, but are seldom predictive, so you don't need to worry about them being repeated in your waking life. However, they do point to unexpressed harmful undercurrents within yourself that urgently need to be faced and understood before they derail you in waking life.

The feeling you experience or wake up with is crucial. If a dream scenario arouses a particular negative emotion, it is doing this because this is a repressed or hidden emotion you need to understand how to manage in your waking life.

WORK

Dreams that have work-related themes typically reflect how you feel others perceive you or how you are performing in your professional life.

Jobs are closely linked to self-esteem in waking life, so the type of job in your dream and your approach to it can be indicators of your current feelings of self-worth and the success or failure of your approach.

The workplace is a centre of learning, anxiety and ambition, so if your dream places you there, it could be suggesting that you are losing your sense of identity and need to find out who you are independent of the role of employee, boss or worker.

A common work-related dream is one in which you have committed a career-ending blunder. This dream isn't urging you to change careers or a sign you are in the wrong career, it is strongly urging you to not get all your identity from your work or status.

If your dream plunges you into a career that isn't your own, consider the skills associated with that career, as your dreaming mind may be urging you to apply those skills or associations to your current waking situation. For example, if you dream you are a nurse, do you need to practise greater self-care? If you dream you are an artist, would a more creative approach be the remedy to a problem?

WRITING

If handwriting is a feature in the dream, remember graphologists study handwriting to learn things about a person's character. What does your dream handwriting reveal about you?

And if you are writing in your dream, consider why your dreaming mind chose that symbol instead of speech to communicate to you, as speech is more direct. Do you need more time to reflect or to formalize something important for your personal growth?

You might want to write down on a piece of paper what you were writing or reading in your dream, as this may well trigger associations.

And what are you writing with? Is it erasable like a pencil or is it a permanent marker? Either way, your dreaming mind has curated this dream symbol for a reason.

MAKING CONNECTIONS

SEEING THE PATTERN

If you have been recording your dreams but still struggle to detect a familiar or returning theme, you could try this exercise:

Give yourself a few moments to review your dream journal. As you look back at your dreams, select three that feel the most memorable and vivid.

Now look for a connecting theme or question between those three dreams. Trust the process. You will find a theme or question.

When you do, ask yourself if the way you are currently reacting to that theme or question is in your best interests or blocking your progress.

The key here is finding some kind of pattern in your dreams, because often simply recognizing there is a pattern is enough to shift it and to start looking for solutions in other ways. Every time you recognize a pattern, you begin to understand yourself better and therein lies the healing purpose of dreams, because when you understand yourself better, you make better decisions for yourself and others. In short, you understand that the power to transform your life lives in *you*.

Above all, though, recurring dream themes are united in their desire to encourage you to get your validation from the inside out rather than the outside in. They tend to happen when external happenings in your waking life are dictating your mood or your internal landscape. You have given away your personal power to forces outside your control. The only way to regain control is to understand that nothing external can define you. The ability to choose – and find – inner calm and peace is always there within you.

Waking up with dream recall on your mind is your daily reminder of your own ability to choose what and who you attract into your life.

CLOSE ENCOUNTERS

Your dreams dramatize your inner conflicts in spectacularly creative ways. If you are recording your dreams on waking, you may at this stage start to notice not just repeating themes, but one recurring message from your deep.

And that overpowering message may be that in some area of your waking life your creative energy is being dissipated. It is being diminished by the expectations of others or by voices from your past that aren't relevant to your current situation. And the purpose of every single one of your dreams is to help you identify, understand and reclaim your own lost power, independence and creative energy.

Try this dream healing exercise right now. Be warned: it requires you to do some improvisation and to use your voice. However, if you prefer to avoid the amateur dramatics you can do it in your head. It is the principle that I am trying to establish here. This is a technique modified from Gestalt dreaming therapy, founded by German psychiatrist and psychoanalyst Fritz Perls.

Choose a recent dream or dream memory from your dream journal and select a key symbol from that dream. For example, if you had a dream where you were drowning, the key symbol is drowning. Now think about the drowning and whether it was in a lake, the sea or a puddle.

Then sit down on a chair if you are not already seated and place another chair in front of you.

Study the chair in front of you and imagine that the director of the dream movie you experienced is sitting right in front of you. Then out loud or in your mind ask the director to explain to you the reason for the drowning scene.

If you can, get up and sit in the opposite chair after you have asked the question, and once sitting in the chair, say the first thing that comes into your mind in response. It doesn't matter how outlandish. This is your dream movie, after all.

Then switch chairs again and continue the conversation until you have some understanding of the context for your dream drowning.

Although this may sound very far-fetched, you have nothing to lose and everything to gain from giving it a go. When you do, you may just find that you surprise yourself. What you are effectively doing is entering into a genuine dialogue with your inner conflict, going right to the heart of the matter or the centre of your inner world to come to a healing resolution.

It might take a few different dream images and attempts for you to really feel the healing power of this exercise, but even if you don't feel you have had a breakthrough, it is a great place to start. If your dialogue involves tension and conflict, you will be showing yourself that there is conflict within you. And whenever there is inner conflict, there is unhappiness.

What you experience in your inner world is often what you attract in your outer world, too. As long as you feel fear, guilt, anger and so on inside, that is what you will encounter and in some cases project onto others and the world.

Dream work zeroes in on all the parts of yourself, and most especially those shadow or hidden parts that your conscious mind often refuses to acknowledge because they make you feel uncomfortable. However, it is those hidden aspects of yourself that are triggering the conflict. They need to be identified, understood and brought into the revealing and healing light of day.

There are many schools of dream therapy and all of them have their merits, but regarding your dreams as dramatizations of your inner conflicts, as Gestalt first proposed, and giving your dream symbols a chance to 'talk' to you is a radical starting-point.

If it doesn't work for you, though, don't let that concern you. Just keep recalling and recording and trusting your dreams and have no doubt that the optimum and deeply personal way to decode them will happen naturally for you.

For further help in finding your own dream way, read on.

THE WORLD CONSPIRING AGAINST YOU

You are likely to have had recurring dream scenarios in which it seems everything and everyone is working against you –

you're running late, missing a train, losing your ticket, unprepared for an exam, facing unexpected obstacles, having phones malfunction and familiar objects vanish, forgetting your lines on stage, arriving late, being unable to find a toilet, failing to impress or graduate, and so on. In these dreams, the overriding theme is that despite your own frantic efforts, nothing is working or is as it should be.

With your growing understanding of dream work, you may gradually begin to understand that these dreams are clearly dramatizing your struggle to impress anyone and everyone except yourself. They are all about not paying attention to what you truly want or need.

When you have these kinds of 'events conspiring against you' dreams, after ruling out that your dreaming mind is being literal and is warning you to be better prepared, the next step is to go deeper. Don't just settle for the dominant theme of delegating your power to others at the expense of yourself; try to be more specific and find out to what, where or whom your energy has been delegated. You need to identify not just why, but in what area of your life this is happening. Then, armed with the detail, you can start making positive changes.

Dreaming of something going terribly wrong doesn't mean it will or is even likely to, however realistic that dream may feel on waking. Your dreaming mind takes you to the brink of failure, rejection and loss to help you not just experience your worst fears, but also to connect you to the resilience – the fighting spirit – that witnessing worst-case scenarios can ignite within you.

And this is yet another reminder for all your dream work: don't settle for a generalized interpretation, go for the personal and be specific. A dream correctly decoded won't paralyse you with uncertainty, it will inspire you to take action and do something positive about a situation that is causing roadblocks and/or anxiety in your waking life.

Be prepared to disappoint others, though, when you listen to your own dreams and find the courage to make positive changes. They will have got used to you operating in a way that suits their expectations. And be prepared for feelings of uncertainty in yourself, too. Change can feel scary but, to risk repeating myself, happiness is never found in your comfort zone. You need to get comfortable feeling uncomfortable. So, the next time you wake up from a dream feeling shaken, don't get anxious, get excited because it signals a big learning curve is about to happen in your life. New revelations are on the horizon.

To recap: Whenever roadblock-scenario dreams start presenting themselves to you, ask yourself what external factors are sucking your energy and/or what inner voice is sabotaging your chances of happiness. In almost all cases, allowing your emotions to flow through you and give you their wisdom will empower you and help you identify what areas of your life need to be reclaimed.

And then?

SAVE YOUR OWN DAY

Hopefully as you read and work through this book and apply the techniques, recurring 'problem' dreams will become less frequent – because in your waking life you have a more experimental approach – and 'saved the day' dreams filled with new symbols and scenarios will start happening more and more. This is because you will be becoming acutely aware of the existence of a powerful inner world – a world of infinite mystery, creativity, intuition and adventure, a world of infinite self-discovery, wisdom, healing and revelation, independent of the expectations of others and the demands of the material world, a world that is in fact your real essence. Your dreams are the portal to your inner power, the part of you that nobody can ever take away from you.

The more conscious you become of your inner power, and the more you desire to be authentic and to avoid conforming to the narratives of others and those within you that no longer serve your best interests, the more empowered you feel. I'm biased, but I believe dream work is your fast pass to the treasure within yourself, to truly being and loving being yourself.

Within you and revealed through the symbolism of your dreams is everything you need to know for healing and personal growth. The simple truth is that when you refuse to acknowledge the existence of these inner resources, you can expect recurring frustrating and 'world conspiring against you' dream themes.

And if the inside-out nature of those dreams isn't understood or acted on, there is every chance of those dreams morphing into full-blown nightmares...

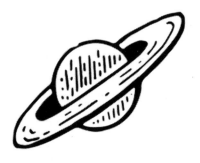

DREAMING IN YOUR DARKNESS

Night light: Without darkness, there is no light, and without light, there is no darkness. Nightmares can be your light when all other lights go out.

Nightmares are surrounded by myths, most of which have their origin in horror movies. They aren't always caused by extreme trauma and abuse. They aren't down to a split personality or an evil spirit. Eating cheese late at night doesn't trigger them. Yes, children are prone to them, but adults can have lots of them too.

And nightmares aren't the same as night terrors.

Night terrors typically happen in the non-REM deep sleep state and involve one recurring symbol of falling, dying, being crushed or other symbols of doom. There may be accompanying physical actions and literal screams. The person may experience hallucinations and/or the feeling of something heavy sitting on their chest – could this be an explanation for so-called incubus and succubus night demon attacks or alien abduction memories?

It's best not to wake a person in this state, but to make sure they are safe in their bed. If they do wake, comfort them until they fall back asleep, as the night terror is unlikely to return and more often than not the next morning the person will have no memory of the episode.

Night terrors often occur during times of extreme stress and change and are more common in childhood. They are related to a disruption in the sleeping and waking process and often resolve themselves, but it is important to seek help from a doctor or sleep therapist if they occur on a frequent basis.

As far as interpreting any dream memories that accompany a night terror, they will be so slight it is best to let them go and focus on dreams that occur before or after them.

Nightmares, on the other hand, occur during the REM stage of sleep, typically the last one before waking, and involve a series of distressing night visions, such as being chased or attacked, and so on. The dreamer clearly remembers them on waking. In many cases the dreams are triggered by unacknowledged guilt and fear and a belief that the dreamer must have done something wrong. Like any other dream, the purpose of them is to help the dreamer recalibrate back to awareness that their true nature is whole. To understand they are good enough, just as they are.

Personal growth happens when you escape the safety net of the comfort zone, and nightmare adventures will inevitably be outside that zone. Nightmares therefore are not to be feared, but embraced as a sign of personal growth.

The biggest myth about nightmares is that they are damaging and should be feared. Quite the opposite: they may make you feel uncomfortable, but they offer remarkable transformative opportunities. Just as a fever indicates an infection is easing, think of your nightmares as a sign that you are healing from within.

SHADOW DREAMING

Your shadow, according to Jungian psychology, is the part of yourself that contradicts the person you think you are, or the persona you present to others, in your waking life. Things you consider unacceptable and feel you need to deny are locked away during the day in your shadow, but they come out to play in your nightmares.

The problem is, these aspects of yourself are a part of you and have a pressing need to be acknowledged and understood.

You can't escape from them or distract yourself from them with a busy schedule. To quote Milton's *Paradise Lost*, 'Which way I fly is Hell, myself am Hell'. The shadow inside, you take it everywhere with you.

Until your shadow is shown the light of day and painful feelings are embraced as important lessons that are part of the rich fabric of your life, your dreams will continue to present them to you time and time again in nightmare symbolism.

Any attempt at consciously repressing or hiding these feelings during the day results in them savagely unleashing their energy at night in your dreams, when your conscious mind lets go of its grip. The more you deny in waking life, the more you feed your shadow, enabling it to claim the throne in the land of your dreams.

A good starting-point when you recognize symbols of your shadow surfacing in your dreams is to show them compassion. These repressed aspects of your personality simply want to be acknowledged. Chances are your dreaming mind has been trying to alert you to something in gentler ways before, but you just haven't reacted. So, it sends a truly shocking scenario your way, knowing that when you wake up, the memory will make you feel so uncomfortable and confused, you will be likely to reflect on it and try to work out the meaning.

Your dreaming mind is resorting to a dose of tough love on your behalf.

Your dreaming mind always has your best interests at heart. Never forget that when you interpret your dreams, even the ones that terrify you.

You may think that your shadow is composed of entirely negative impulses, such as jealousy, anger, hate, and so on, and while this is commonly the case, it is also the case that you may have learned during childhood to suppress aspects of yourself that aren't toxic. For example, you may have diminished your assertiveness, because your parents or carers didn't approve and back then you needed their approval to feel loved and nurtured. When you become an adult, though, there is no longer any need to suppress who you truly are.

When aspects of yourself that are creative and empowering are hidden, you can meet them in your dreams in what is termed the 'golden' shadow. But whether you meet your dark or golden shadow in slumberland, the opportunity for transformation is unsurpassed.

Nightmares are so shocking and disturbing, you have absolutely no choice but to recall them. Your dreaming mind is presenting you quite literally with a 'grow or die' ultimatum. If you want to avoid the nightmare and the distressing fear blocking your progress in waking life, you have to reflect on the meaning and give your shadow a chance to be noticed. When that recognition occurs, and you face your fear and start to enter into a meaningful dialogue with your shadow, chances are you'll find that the fear dissipates. In the words of Jung, 'Where your fear is, there is your task.'

Just as there is darkness (night) and there is light (day), and you can't have one without the other, there is a positive and a negative impulse within us all. Inner strength isn't denying or hiding the presence of the negative (that's toxic positivity), but being aware that the potential for darkness lives within you and knowing that you are the one in control of which aspects of your personality you decide to give your energy to. You always have the power to choose to do the healthiest thing. Feelings don't just happen to you – you let them in.

And when you do acknowledge your shadow, you might just find it is full of surprises and has much of value to teach you. Seeds grow in the dark. The beauty of a lotus flower emerges from muddy waters.

Coming to terms with your own shadow – and how in your waking life problems emerge when you project it onto others – can give you self-awareness, along with a dose of vitality, motivation and humility – all the things you might need to become a fulfilled human being. It is ironic that often the emotions you deny the most are the ones that, once understood, can completely elevate you.

Above all, nightmares encourage curiosity about what triggers them, and curiosity is the catalyst for dream decoding and personal growth. Simply thinking about a nightmare can bring hope into your life. A nightmare has a sense of urgency that other dreams don't, and that urgency is real. Something in your waking consciousness must shift, now. You are being called to expand and evolve. Typically, that shift will be in your own mindset or perspective, the way you speak to and judge yourself. Make sure that the way you speak to yourself is always compassionate.

FACING YOURSELF IN THE MIRROR

You may have heard of mirror-work techniques to deal with the imbalances and insecurities in your waking life that often express themselves in nightmare symbols. In mirror work you remove the projection from others and ask yourself how what is happening outside you reflects what is happening within you. For example, if someone criticizes you, stare long and hard in the mirror and ask how you are criticizing yourself.

Mirror work can be a revelation, but it only leads to personal growth if you connect to the inner healer, not the inner critic. Leave connecting to and releasing your inner critic to the wisdom of your dreaming mind. When awake, whenever you look at yourself in the mirror, focus not on inner reproach but on what is special about you. A simple way to start doing that is to stare into the beautiful, utterly unique whirlpools of mystery that are your own eyes. And when you gaze into your own eyes, be sure to think of them as 'the windows to your soul', aka your dreams.

CLASSIC NIGHTMARES

Just as your dreams are personal, your nightmares are too, and what is terrifying to one dreamer may not be to another, but here are some dream symbols you have met before in this book which can take on additional nightmarish qualities. If they do, you are strongly advised to pay close attention. In other words, don't ignore any dream, most especially these.

ANIMAL ATTACK

Wild animals attacking or chasing you can be utterly terrifying. This is because animals in dreams are your instinctual drives, demanding your attention.

BURIAL

Creepy dreams of being buried alive can signal feeling trapped without a lifeline. You must find a way to escape restrictions and express yourself and ask for help and support.

DEATH AND DYING

If death and dying – or related symbols, such as coffins and graveyards – feature in a dream, even if the setting isn't frightening it can feel very much like a nightmare when you wake up, especially if you yourself and/or a loved one die in the dream. Your first instinct is likely to be panic that this might be a premonition or warning of some kind. Time to set the record straight, especially as this is one of the most commonly reported dream themes.

Dying to live

The overwhelming majority of dreams about death and dying aren't precognitions. As almost all of us have had this kind of dream at some point in our lives, if they were, there would be plenty of evidence to draw on, and we haven't got that evidence. All we have are some exceedingly rare cases when dreams of someone dying have come true, but there are always other considerations and elements in the dream which didn't play out. So, the rule of thumb is to consider death in dreams as a metaphor.

Your dreaming heart resorts to the symbolism of death when it has tried and failed to send you the same message in gentler symbolic ways, such as flowers wilting or sunshine instantly transforming to snow. And the message it wants to send you is that something meaningful in your life is ending. This could be the feelings you have for someone or the feelings they have for you, or it could be a mindset that is dying within you. But the good news is that with every dream death there is always a new beginning waiting in the wings.

Most of us fear death greatly because it is the great unknown, but your dreaming mind is taking you there to help you process your feelings about it and at the same time connecting you to a spiritual force within you that can transcend your material body, time and space, and perhaps even death.

Should you die in your own dream or be in the process of dying, this is a potent symbol of change or an ending happening within your life, or one that needs to happen for your well-being. Focus on the manner of that death. Is it something natural or something imposed on you by outside forces, for example are you murdered? If you are killed in your dream this indicates you may be feeling pressured by others to change or transform something. If you do the killing/murdering your dreaming mind wants you to end something, typically a mindset that is dragging you down. Your dreaming mind uses this shocking scenario to wake you up to the importance of taking stock of your life and making positive changes. Indeed, dreams of your own death are among the most transformative, as they suggest that your unconscious is beyond ready to let go of mindsets and personas or roles in your waking life that may have served you in the past but have now become roadblocks to your happiness.

Such a dream can also remind you that death and life are intertwined, and if you fear death, you also fear life. Focus not on endings, but on the joyful discovery of new aspects of consciousness waiting for you to grow into them.

If the person dying or dead in your dream is not you but a loved one, this is likely to feel like a nightmare. But now that you know dreams reflect what is currently happening in your life, it is time to get down to the honest business of decoding.

This dream may suggest that the relationship you have with the dying or dead person is changing, or has to change for the sake of the relationship. Perhaps you or they are moving on to another stage in life, or you need to change a certain opinion you have about them. Parents, for example, often dream about children dying when they leave home and panic it may be a premonition. It isn't. The dream is stating that the childhood phase of their relationship is ending, but with every ending there is always a new beginning and here it is the birth of an adult relationship with their children.

If you do dream of the death of a loved one, brainstorm how that relationship can be improved with a change of mindset or routine or a fresh start in some way.

Should someone you know of but have never met, like a celebrity, die in your dream, think about the first thing you associate with that person. Your dreaming mind will want you to apply that association to your personal growth and to reflect on whether it needs to be released or reconsidered in some way.

And should a stranger die in a dream, this again is symbolic of something in your waking life that you are losing touch with.

Dream bereavements spotlight the power of change in your waking life and the draining consequences of trying to stop time or hold back change or keep your mind closed, resulting in a kind of 'living death'. A closed mind, like a parachute that won't open mid-flight, is 'deadly'. For many of us, death is our greatest fear, because it remains the great unknown. However, when you understand that connecting to your inner world and your dreams can help you accept that fear and delve deeply into it, and that death is just a part of the miracle of life, this is a priceless opportunity for you to be reborn, as you are every single morning when you wake up.

DROWNING

Dreaming that you are drowning is a clear sign that you are letting your feelings make decisions for you in your waking life. Your dreaming mind is sharply encouraging you to manage your emotions better and showcasing just how destructive it is for you on an emotional and psychological level to repress hidden feelings.

There is some area in your waking life where you are refusing to allow the natural flow, and if you continue to do that, your emotions will at some point overwhelm or 'drown' you. During the day you may have become accustomed to rationalizing or suppressing your emotions, but that isn't possible in your dreams, where you may find yourself hit by a tidal wave of unconscious emotion.

INJURY

Dreams in which you are injured can symbolize a desire to escape the responsibilities and burdens of life. They also suggest that you urgently need to let go of some mindset or situation or relationship in your waking life that is draining your life-force.

NATURAL DISASTERS

These frightening dreams can signal personal problems in danger of raging out of control. Your dreaming mind feels it is unacceptable and impossible for you to continue to ignore them.

PARALYSIS

Being paralysed or unable to move or speak in a dream can suggest that you are feeling stifled from taking on too much responsibility. Sometimes you have to make a decision to move forward, even if that decision isn't the perfect one.

Sleep paralysis is a natural state that happens when you enter REM sleep. Your body is not only unable to move in this state, but there is also an absence of stress hormones, which means that you experience nightmare scenarios without harmful stress hormones being released. However, dreaming of being unable to move or speak isn't a symbolic reference to sleep paralysis. Your dreaming mind is using this symbolism to alert you to something or someone paralysing you in your waking life. Sometimes this will be a person you know or a situation you are in, but more often than not the paralysis has an inside source. Conflicting parts of your personality – your desire to break free and your desire to stay safe, for example – are leaving you unable to move in any direction.

Paralysis is the enemy of personal growth, which is all about forward momentum, so this dream is urging you to deal with whatever it is that is trapping you from the inside out or outside in before the paralysis takes over and destroys your chances of happiness.

PLANE, TRAIN OR CAR CRASHES

If you find yourself dreaming about an out-of-control vehicle, this suggests that events in your waking life risk spiralling out of control. It is imperative that you get in the driver's seat or, if you are the driver, that you drive more skilfully.

PROPERTY DAMAGE

Your home represents your inner world, so if you dream your house is on fire or damaged or destroyed, it suggests a lack of self-care or some form of self-sabotage. Your emotional life is in danger.

On the flip side, if you dream of finding new rooms in your home or doing home improvements, some aspect of your inner life is on the mend.

How to decode your nightmares

On waking from a nightmare with disturbing and distressing images and feelings, first of all do some deep breathing to slow your pulse and heart rate down. Breathe in calm and understanding and breathe out anxiety and fear. You are safe in your bed, but there's no denying your dreaming mind is screaming for attention. You need to process that.

Respect your dreaming mind and write down the key words and feelings of the nightmare without judging or trying to make sense of it.

Then, having reassured your dreaming mind you will reflect on the nightmare later, let go of it and go back to sleep, or get up if your day is starting.

Later in the day, find a few minutes of calm and quiet and revisit the nightmare in your journal.

Then rescript it so that there is a positive ending. You can do this by writing it down in your journal or through visualization. It doesn't matter how, just make sure you do it, because this will make it clear to your conscious and unconscious mind that you are in control. You have the power to transform your inner demons into inner angels. Use your power with great responsibility.

Writing down your nightmares and rescripting them will often release a surge of creativity, so celebrate that transcendent feeling when you notice it rising inside you. Know, too, that nightmares can make great gothic or horror stories. Did you know that without nightmares we might never have had the first sci-fi novel, *Frankenstein*? The plot emerged from a dream Mary Shelley had, and the plot of Robert Louis Stevenson's *Dr Jekyll and Mr Hyde* came from a dream too.

Perhaps your nightmare oyster contains similar creative pearls. Or perhaps it will do something just as magical and unlock creativity within you on a personal level. Writing down your dreams is a fantastic creativity hack if you ever experience writer's or creative block, because you are connecting to the part of your brain that is intuitive and creative.

Then, when you have rescripted your nightmare and reminded yourself nightmares don't happen to you but for you, start brainstorming the meaning of the dream symbols. Emphasis on the word *symbols*. Your nightmares are not literal. They are using horrific symbolism to help you rid yourself of inner hostility, the drive for perfection and the energy within you that is locked or tied up in all that. Your dreaming mind – your best friend – wants you to release that energy so it can be used positively in your waking life.

HOW TO REDUCE YOUR RISK OF NIGHTMARES

Knowing that nightmares are transformative gifts, my first question is: why would you want to?

However, if nightmares are interfering with your sleep, this isn't good news for your holistic health, so here are some practical things you can do:

- Avoid eating large meals late at night or drinking alcohol. Digestion while you are asleep heats up your body and prevents you getting a restful night, and when your sleep is fitful, the chance of nightmares increases. Alcohol is a toxin for your body, brain and soul, and the dreams it triggers will be as hallucinatory as the substance itself.

- Steer clear of watching horror and/or gory movies right before bedtime, when your brain is relaxed and receptive. Remember your brain draws on what you think, feel, do and experience in the day, and especially last thing before sleep, to create its dream symbols.

⊚ Be sure to reduce your stress levels during the day and rule out the possibility of night terrors and sleep or medical disorders too. Your doctor should always be your first port of call if anything is seriously impacting the quality of your sleep and your health and well-being.

In short, all the quality sleep rules covered in Lesson 1 will help you keep nightmares at bay, as will your belief that a dream-catcher hung over your bed or a protective crystal placed on your bedside table or moon water drunk during the day can enhance your chances of sweet dreams.

But the best nightmare cure is to diligently do your dream work. Follow the recall and decoding advice in this book, as it will help you lose your fear of nightmares, and if one springs up, you won't panic. You might even get excited, because you know understanding it can release tremendous creative, healing and psychic energy within you. And you can always rescript your nightmares too.

Willingness to face and embrace things you fear within yourself is essential for personal growth and is what dream work is all about. So, revisiting your dream demons to see what they have to teach you is crucial. In the world of your dreams it is damaging to run away from something you fear. The only way to escape is to go in deep and to be *changed* by that experience.

Regrettably, we have a tendency to wake up in a nightmare at its most terrifying point, depriving ourselves of the opportunity to fully face, understand and go into our fear within the dream. This can be done in waking life through brainstorming your nightmares, but if it can be done in the dreaming state – and if you can train yourself to stay with the dream and know you are dreaming – all the better. This is called lucid dreaming. (More about this rare but natural and wildly promising dream state and how you can trigger it yourself in the final lesson.)

THE TIDES OF CHANGE

Night after night, your dreams are identifying areas of your life or your mindset that urgently need to recalibrate. But you can't solve today's problems with the mindset that created them. And sometimes even the wrong change is better than no change, because it will force you to experience and, in the process, learn. As contradictory as it may sound, your dreaming mind prefers you to fail and fail again than to stand still. Life, both with your eyes wide open and wide shut, is an endless flow, so fail often and learn fast.

Trust your dreams. They are important messages being delivered to you from your own soul.

PSYCHIC DREAMS

When you lose your fear of your inner world and encountering both the angels and the demons that linger there, you may find that you start to experience another special category of dreams – psychic dreams.

Indeed, I have found over the years that dream work and psychic awakening often go hand in hand. This is because dream work helps you understand yourself better, make better decisions in your waking life and grow in self-confidence. And the more self-confident you are, the more your innate psychic abilities flower.

Believe it or not, we are all born with a sixth sense. It is in our DNA. We have just forgotten how to notice it and, most important of all, believe in it. The only difference between people who say they are psychic and those who don't think they are is that those who say they are believe they are. It is exactly the same with dream work: believe that your dreams have precious wisdom for you and they will deliver.

Interestingly, if those who say they aren't psychic, because they value logic and reason more than intuition, commit to meditation practices for a few weeks, brain scans show that the dreaming parts of their brain fire up. And when they fire up, often the psychic dreams that come through are clearer than those of people who are more sensitive.

So, we all have transcendent potential within. To access that potential, you simply need to notice, understand and believe in it. Students of dreams know the inner world is where all their psychic powers are born.

I think it is a mistake to divide dreams into 'psychic' and 'non-psychic', as they all transcend time and space and offer illumination. Having said that, though, some dreams seem to be pointing more clearly towards a psychic definition than others. Here are the main categories that I have identified from my research – and if you notice any of them, write them down in your dream journal alongside all your other amazing dreams. Treat all your dreams as endorsements of your inner magic.

AFTERLIFE COMMUNICATION DREAMS

Throughout my career as a writer on dreams and spiritual topics, I have lost count of the number of afterlife dreams that have been sent to me. These dreams fall into a special category of their own. They are often intensely vivid and memorable and stand apart from other symbolic dreams in that they typically have a beginning, a middle and an end (symbolic dreams are often like fragments where you find yourself in the middle rather than the beginning of the story). They also feel *über*-realistic; the departed loved one is instantly recognizable and appears in a familiar setting such as the dreamer's bedroom. The dreamer wakes up feeling as if they have actually spoken to someone on the other side and they don't feel sad that it wasn't 'real'. Quite the opposite.

I know I said I wouldn't share other people's dreams, as they tend not to be relatable, but in this case, if you haven't yet had an afterlife communication dream, I want to share this one, messaged to me by Dawn, to give you pause for thought:

> I was on the edge of sleep, or perhaps I was asleep, I'm not sure, but suddenly a clear image of my recently departed mum burst through. She was sitting with her back to me on a park bench, one she used to sit on a lot when she was alive. I knew it was her and she turned around and smiled, beckoning for me to sit on the bench beside her.
>
> When I was sitting next to her, she started talking to me. I can't recall all the words, but I know I heard my name and the names of my children. She looked so vibrant. At one point I think I opened my eyes, but she wasn't there in

the darkness of night. I closed my eyes again and was back on the bench with my mum. After that, I kept my eyes tightly shut. I wanted to capture this living connection with her for as long as I could.

The next morning when I woke up, I closed my eyes and returned in my mind's eye to that bench – and every time I miss my mum or get tearful, I return again to it. It doesn't feel as real as that first dream, but the memory of it sustains me immensely.

In some cultures, the dream world is considered to be a portal or a door to the afterlife and it seems that it might just be.

Dreams – like our lives – are an infinite mystery, so perhaps they are a place where the departed can drop in to offer reassurance to us that they are still alive within our hearts and souls, and always will be.

It is often said people die twice, the first time physically and the second time when they are forgotten, so afterlife communication dreams keep your departed loved ones alive within you.

Much depends on whether or not you believe the afterlife is real. However, regardless of belief, research shows that in over 90 per cent of cases, these kinds of dreams are incredibly therapeutic for the grieving. The dreamer doesn't wake up distressed, but comforted. They have an understanding that death ends a life, not a relationship.

Never fear conversations with departed loved ones in your dreams. They are your dreaming mind helping you process grief and keeping your loved ones alive within your heart.

Psychologists argue that these dreams are simply the grieving brain processing the trauma of loss, but if that were always the case, nightmares would be far more likely than a comforting dream scenario. These dreams feel spirit sent.

DREAM WORKING

If in your waking life you are a caring and compassionate person, you don't stop being that person when you dream, and you may find yourself in the role of spiritual helper in a dream. For example, you may dream you are there when someone is dying and in need of a spiritual presence, or you may find yourself dreaming of helping others through traumas.

If you believe we are non-physical beings whose consciousness isn't limited by the body, then it makes sense that when we dream, our consciousness doesn't just help and heal ourselves, but is of service to others too. So, if you wake up from a good night's sleep feeling a little tired and you have no health issues, perhaps you have been a busy spiritual force for others in your sleep!

DREAMS OF UNBORN CHILDREN

Many parents have messaged me over the years to say they met their future children in their dreams, sometimes before they were born or even thought about.

I have personal experience of this in that I met my son in my dreams when I was not married, dating or even thinking about settling down and getting pregnant. In that dream I was struggling to climb a mountain and a hand appeared to help me. It was the hand of an Asian boy with the deepest brown eyes and a round face with a tiny mole. Years later I recognized that face, those eyes and that tiny mole when my son became a toddler.

PAST-LIFE DREAMS

These dreams have been researched as evidence for reincarnation, the theory that our souls are reborn time and time again. In some instances, the dreamer wakes up with memories from a former life that they could not possibly know and which later prove to be correct. Add to that the fact that some of these past-life dreamers are children, and the psychic dream plot thickens.

PRECOGNITIVE DREAMS

Perhaps this has happened to you at some point: you are going about your day as normal and then suddenly something or someone reminds you of a dream you had. You've been there before in your dreams. Often, this won't be something major, but something trivial. For example, you may dream of an item of jewellery and then the next day see one of your colleagues wearing exactly the same item of jewellery for the first time.

When this happens to you, make note. Record it as data in your dream journal. Even though the *déjà rêvé* – 'already dreamed' – moment may be trivial, your dreaming mind has drawn your attention to that symbol for a reason. Brainstorm the meaning as normal, but with the awareness that the course-correcting potential of this moment in time is being highlighted in bold for you.

In waking life, your brain is always making connections to help you accurately sense the future. Your body provides you with symptoms, for example raised heart rate and feelings in your gut. This is called presentiment. So, remember to check in with your body on waking to see if that triggers more dream recall. And if you can sense the future when you are awake, you can sense it in your dreams. Indeed, the majority of precognitive experiences happen in the dreaming state.

The phenomenon of precognitive dreaming is where I believe the future of dream research lies. All dreams are potentially precognitive in that they preview potential futures to offer you choices about the future you are creating in your present. In other words, your dreams are giving you a threat rehearsal, warning or information to help you make better choices about an upcoming turning-point in your life.

Again, since dreams allow your consciousness to move beyond time, space, life and death, keep your mind open here. Never rule out the possibility that they can take you back into your past and forward into your future, sometimes at the same time!

SHARED DREAMS

These are when one person has a dream and the very same night someone they are close to in waking life has a very similar dream. This is most likely to happen to siblings, spouses and close friends.

If this happens to you and a loved one, it can make for a deeply fascinating discussion the next morning. The idea that you can meet someone in your dreams opens up all sorts of extraordinary conversations.

TELEPATHIC DREAMS

Dreams in which you the dreamer see, feel or experience what is happening to someone else are more common and natural than you may think. They typically happen to people who are super-close, such as family members and loved ones, but in rare cases they can involve friends and colleagues or sometimes people you barely know.

Should this kind of dream happen to you, be sure to record it, as it is proving to you that you are a psychic dreamer. It's always best to assume a dream is symbolizing your mindset first, but if you believe it's about another person, keep a record of it so that you have proof and that over time you can recognize when these kinds of telepathic/empathetic dreams happen.

EMPOWER YOUR PSYCHIC DREAMS

You don't have to believe in psychic powers to decode your dreams. All you need to do is keep your mind open, as this will help you tune into your hidden potential and avoid doubt and scepticism taking over.

Recording your dreams and understanding the themes that occur can help you identify when a dream seems to be even more psychic than usual. Your personal sense of the dream is key. Trust your inner psychic, but ask as many questions of your psychic dreams as any other dreams.

Dreams that don't come true have just as much to teach you as those that do, because every dream is an authentic reflection of your current mindset and situations in your waking life. In this way, every dream is potentially precognitive, because what you currently feel, think and do in your waking life is the future you are busy creating.

This is another reminder that simply thinking about the meaning of your dreams can change your life, and in the case of nightmares, if you don't like what you glimpse, the dream has offered you an opportunity to course correct and avoid the future you are hurtling towards *if* you continue feeling, thinking and doing the same as you are now. In this way, your dreams are always showcasing both your present and your potential future. The future is out there, but you – yes, you – have the inner power to change it.

THE DARKNESS BEFORE YOUR DAWN

You head into darkness every night, simply by falling asleep. You probably don't give any thought to it, because it just happens. From now on I want you to reflect on how you do it every night.

Why? Consider the Pirahã tribe from Brazil, who have been described as the happiest people on Earth. They are a simple people who base their values on relationships and, it seems, lack of sleep. They tend to nap rather than sleep, because they believe sleeping is a risk. You can't protect yourself from snakes when you are deeply asleep. This makes sense to a primitive culture, but not to a society that has evolved to ensure snakes don't attack at night. I'm most certainly not suggesting that you nap instead of sleep – a good night's sleep is crucial for your dream work – but I do want to draw your attention to a belief the Pirahã have about sleep.

They believe that if you fall asleep for more than a few hours, you wake up no longer being you anymore. Pirahã who sleep longer than planned refer to the person they were before their sleep as a different person. They use the term 'him' or 'her' rather than 'me' when referencing their past. And they have an intuitive point here, as every time you go to sleep at night you are regenerating.

Contrary to popular belief, your body and brain don't rest when you sleep. Your cells renew and your brain adds knowledge to your store of unconscious knowledge and explores all current options for you in the world of your dreams.

It is up to you whether you wake up each morning a more aware, evolved version of yourself than you were the day before. The more curious you are and the more you learn and reflect during the day, the more you will evolve while you are sleeping. Each night when you fall asleep, the person you were that day metaphorically 'dies'. You are born anew physically, mentally, emotionally and spiritually every morning.

What a life-affirming and dream-empowering thought.

FALLING ASLEEP

So, this evening when it is time to retire, don't just flop into bed without thinking about the profound significance of what you are about to do. Treat the act of preparing to go to sleep and entering the world of dreams with the reverence it deserves. Perform this bedtime ritual:

> Sit on your bed, close your eyes and slow down your breath until you can count to three on each inhale and

three on each exhale. As you do this, straighten your spine, relax your shoulders, release the tension in your face (many of us frown constantly or tense our facial muscles without realizing it) and lower your chin slightly.

When you feel comfortable and relaxed, lengthen your exhale count to four and then to six, all the while keeping the inhale on three counts. When you are comfortably inhaling on three and exhaling on six, consciously let go of the day with gratitude on each exhale, and on each inhale, allow the restorative and healing power of your breathing to welcome in the regenerative sleep and illuminating dreaming that are sure to follow.

Allow around five to ten minutes for this deep sleep ritual, and when you feel sleepy, gently lie down on your bed. Turn the lights off and close your eyes, without checking any devices, especially your phone! Focus your thoughts and feelings on the dreams that are sure to come.

If this was your last day and you didn't wake up in the morning, would you feel at peace with who you are and what you have achieved? How would you be remembered? What would your obituary say? If you don't like what you think it might say, count your blessings, because tonight you get to dream new dreams and tomorrow is another day. Let tomorrow be a day when your intuition guides and inspires you to be the best that you can be.

The human race has existed for millions of years and we still don't know why we are here or why we wake up each new morning. What is clear, though, is that each morning we wake up with the opportunity to learn anew and this is a miracle we take for granted too many times.

Another miracle we take for granted is the gift of intuition, which, like an inner GPS, can guide us in the right direction through gut instinct by day and dream messages by night.

Pause for a moment now and let the following dreaming through darkness quotations flow through you. You might want to read them out loud first, so your conscious waking mind and your unconscious dreaming mind work together and get the message loud and clear.

Then revisit page 4 and reflect more deeply than ever before on those dream-work power points.

Even a happy life cannot be without a measure of darkness, and the word 'happy' would lose its meaning if it were not balanced by sadness... The best political, social and spiritual work you can do is to withdraw the projection of your own shadow onto others.

Carl Jung

People are like stained-glass windows. They sparkle and shine when the sun is out, but when the darkness sets in their true beauty is revealed only if there is light from within.

Elisabeth Kübler-Ross

Light is to darkness what love is to fear. In the presence of one, the other disappears.

Marianne Williamson

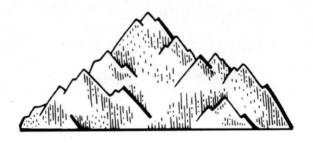

DESIGN YOUR OWN DREAMS

Night light: Just thinking about the meaning of a dream can change and bring healing to your life.

'To sleep, perchance to dream.' No more 'perchance' about it. From now on, you sleep to dream big. The more creative and healing your dreams are, the more creative and fulfilling your waking life will be.

Most of us leave our chances of having healing dreams to chance. We are still of the mindset that dreams just happen to us, but I hope everything in this book has shown you that your dreams are *your* creation.

Knowing your dreams are both a reflection and a trend-setting preview of your waking life, doesn't it make sense to do what you can to influence the contents of your dreams? Why not take matters into your own hands, or dreaming mind, and become your own dreamscaper?

BECOME A DREAMSCAPER

Dreamscaping isn't the same as lucid dreaming, which is becoming aware you are dreaming when you are dreaming. Dreamscaping is creating a dream plan before you go to sleep. For example, if you have had a tough day, before you go to sleep you may ask for a dream that will provide a distraction. Visualize or describe to yourself the opening scene, using your senses. Perhaps you want to fly to the moon, or visit Alaska, or solve a murder. Choose whatever relaxes and energizes you. You are setting the scene here and trusting your dreaming mind will continue the story.

The reason you think about what you want to dream about before you go to sleep is because your brain is highly suggestible then. That is why it is important to go to bed with a calm mind and grateful heart, and never go to bed feeling stressed or arguing.

But is it really possible to plan your dreams?

Research shows that it is possible to decide what you want to dream about before you go to sleep, up to a point. This doesn't mean full control, it means influence. Dreams, like the ocean, can be navigated, but you can never fully control or predict them.

Your ability to skilfully dreamscape will depend on your openness to your inner world, your understanding of dream work and your personal dream themes. Would you like to try it?

Plan your dream

Just before you go to sleep, tell yourself what you want to dream about. Writing down your intention in your dream journal can help, as can writing it on a piece of paper and placing that under your pillow, as sometimes the written word imprints itself onto the unconscious more deeply than thoughts and words alone. Keep your dream plan brief, as your unconscious mind doesn't process or respond to words well – words belong to the waking world.

If you can visualize the dream entry point, do so, Ensure you are physically relaxed and then visualize the scene, really feel it, experience in your mind's eye the colour, the texture, the setting, the sounds of the dream scene before you.

If visualization doesn't come easy to you, search online for a picture that recreates your dream entry point, or draw one yourself. It doesn't matter if you don't consider yourself artistic, just give your dreaming mind a floor plan to work with. And if you want to return to a past dream, because you feel something vital was hidden there for you or because you enjoyed it so much you didn't want it to end, follow the same process.

If you have aphantasia, a condition which limits the ability to visualize, talk to yourself about the dream you are planning, or think about it. Describe it in words or thoughts as if you were a film critic reviewing a movie.

SHOULD YOU TRY TO INFLUENCE YOUR DREAMS?

You may be asking yourself this question, but don't worry, influencing your unconscious mind in a *positive* way is always a good thing.

Why? What you believe about yourself and your life on a deep unconscious level tends to be what you attract or manifest into your life. So, influencing a dream in the direction you want it to go – in other words, seeing yourself doing and saying what you want to, having confidence, and so on, convinces your unconscious that something is really possible for you. And when you believe things are possible for you, everything changes for the better in your waking life.

And if you feel you need guidance, just ask.

ASKING FOR GUIDANCE

You have likely comprehended by now that dream decoding is all about excavating the hidden issue your intuition, your heart, has noticed during the day but your waking, rational mind has buried. Your dreaming mind wants to be in conversation with you about it. So, call on it for guidance before you go to sleep – aka incubating a dream – or ask for more clarity on a previous dream you can't yet understand.

How to ask your dreaming mind for guidance

In many ways, calling on your dreaming mind for guidance is similar to reciting a nightly prayer. You need to find your own unique way to speak to it before you go to sleep, but I strongly advise talking to it with respect at all times and, after you have asked for a specific dream, reassuring it that you want to recall the dream and will record it, for example:

Dear dreaming mind, please send me a dream to help me understand myself and my life better. I will recall my dreams and will write them down on waking. Thank you for your wise guidance.

Thanking your dreaming mind in advance for the guidance you fully expect to receive also strikes an assured note.

On waking, be true to your word and write down any dream memories on your mind, and make a note of how you feel too. Don't stress if the dream seems to have absolutely nothing to do with your request, because more often than not when you reflect on it later in the day, you will find that there is a uniting theme.

When decoding, focus on the key symbol and theme. The devil isn't always in the dream details. In dreams, as in life, often it is the bigger picture you need to focus on to give you a sense of proportion.

By all means ask your dreaming mind to help you get in touch with your inner wisdom and expect it to send you the energy shift or understanding. But don't expect it to wipe away all your troubles; rather, it will shine a light on them to help you understand what you need to forgive or allow within yourself to move forward and make empowering decisions.

There is no area of your waking life you can't ask your dreaming mind for guidance on. Tailor your dream request to include the specifics. The only requirement is that the question you ask your dreaming mind about is one that speaks clearly to your heart.

RELATIONSHIPS

Your heart is the home of all your relationships, and asking your dreaming mind for guidance there will feel natural. Simply ask your dreaming mind to help you understand how you feel about someone in your life or to offer you advice on a specific relationship. Remember to be polite to your dreaming mind and grateful for its guidance.

Know that if you ask your dreaming mind for help with your love life, chances are it will send you dream symbols that can help you find the greatest love of all – yourself. It will remind you that love can't be found outside yourself until you find it within yourself and will encourage you to attract rather than chase love by spotlighting what it is within you that is keeping love and healthy relationships at bay. For example, not feeling worthy of love, being afraid of feeling vulnerable, expecting rejection, and so on. Your dreaming mind wants you to value yourself and fill yourself up with self-respect and self-love before sharing what you have with others.

WORK

Your dreaming mind can also get to work brainstorming your life direction or work or role in life. Again, it won't be an oracle or remove all your problems. But what it will do is reveal to you what will improve the quality of your waking life or make you feel more fulfilled.

You may think being wealthy and popular is the definition of success, but your dreaming mind sees the bigger picture and is only concerned with your inner wealth. Look no further than the vast numbers of wealthy, talented, famous, successful and deeply unhappy people to prove the wisdom of your dreaming mind here. It will drill down on helping you understand that inner peace isn't something you achieve when you are a success, but something that must come *before* success.

Your waking mind: 'I will find inner joy, love and peace when things work out.'

Your dreaming mind: 'When I find inner joy, love and peace, things will work out.'

And if you unconsciously think of yourself in terms of failure, that is what the world will reflect back to you, both in your waking life and your dreams.

The same applies to money and prosperity. If you unconsciously believe you don't deserve to prosper, your dreams will mirror that inner poverty back to you in the hope that you will become aware of it and start creating a shift from within.

Change your dreams, change your life.

PERSONAL GROWTH, SELF-CONFIDENCE

If you value your personal growth, you must treasure your night vision. Every dream is an empowering message from your inner therapist. The journey to self-love and self-reliance is the journey of dream work.

Dreams are symbolic messages from your higher self, reminding you that you are loved. If your dreams are anxiety related, the only thing missing may be your belief in the existence of your higher self.

You can ask your dreaming mind to send you a dream that spotlights the roadblocks to this belief. The reason this is so empowering, and in my opinion the first question to ask your dreaming mind, is that in our waking lives we are often our own worst enemy, unaware that it isn't other people or things that are handicapping us, but ourselves. Being willing to confront aspects within yourself that are holding you back is the royal road to personal growth.

As I mentioned earlier, what you think and feel is what you tend to attract into your life. And those thoughts and feelings are often the result of how you were taught to think and feel by parents or carers, siblings or teachers. They aren't your own beliefs, but ingrained mindsets.

Some of these will be positive, but even if they are, you may have outgrown them. If you have ever heard yourself offer 'That's the way I am' as an explanation, what you are really saying is: 'That's what I believe I am.' Your dreaming mind wants to show you that whatever you believe about yourself doesn't have to be set in stone and become a self-fulfilling prophecy. There's always the opportunity for change. Life *is* change, so if you limit change, you paralyse yourself in both your dreams and your waking life.

Night after night your dreaming mind is doing all it can to show you that you don't have to continue to think or behave in a certain way. Changing your thought and feeling patterns can change and heal your life. The problem is that most of us aren't aware of our negative patterns, and again that's where dream work comes in. Dreams can spotlight all those draining feelings of not being worthy or good enough, those feelings of fear and anger, and the limitations they all place upon you.

And the wonderful thing is that dreams also showcase to you that although your thoughts are powerful, you are the creator of them and infinitely more powerful. Every morning when you wake up, you can change that inner narrative. Every moment is a new beginning. You don't even have to wait until your next dream. You can start right here, right now, in this present moment. Pause for a minute and analyse how you are currently thinking about yourself and whether it makes you feel good. If it isn't making you feel good, why are you choosing to think it? If you ate something once and it made you feel sick, you wouldn't choose to eat it again. Do the same with your waking thoughts. Catch and course correct them as often as you can and notice how your dreaming world mirrors that shift back to you. Indeed, noticing that your dreams feel more energizing and creative is a sure-fire sign of accelerated personal, mental, emotional and spiritual growth.

Don't panic if your dreams aren't there yet. They will be when you're ready. Unless you are Jack, you can't plant a seed and expect a beanstalk to grow overnight. Be patient and trusting with yourself. The more you focus on what you want in your waking life and not on what you don't want, and the more you forgive yourself and release limiting beliefs, the more you will feel empowered from the inside out. Keep experimenting in your waking life and keep dreaming big dreams.

And don't beat yourself up when you make mistakes. Remember, mistakes are opportunities to learn and grow. Problems, remember, are the force and the wind beneath your wings. And whenever you feel broken or empty, it is a sign that you are about to grow. Sometimes growth hurts, but you are about to emerge from the darkness, spiral rather than loop, and see yourself and your life from a higher perspective. Hang in there!

Your dreams are always aiming to get you to a place where you love yourself and can look into your own eyes – the windows to your soul – in a mirror and tell yourself that you are good enough and believe it. Why not find a mirror or camera right now?

Design your Own Dreams

Your eyes have it

Stand or sit in front of a mirror and stare deeply into your own eyes.

   Notice how this makes you feel.

   Notice what thoughts come into your mind.

Looking into your own eyes is perhaps where all your dream-decoding work should really begin. From now on, before you start brainstorming the meaning of any dream you might want to take a moment to look into your own eyes for the love and vision you need to find your answers.

In some ways, dreaming is looking deep into your own eyes every single night. The experience can feel unsettling and electrifying at the same time.

Always keep that sacred respect for your dreams, whatever they reveal to you from the inside out. When you respect and fall in love with decoding your dreams, what you are actually doing is respecting and falling in love with yourself.

And when you feel your dream decoding has identified a theme or made you aware of a mindset that is attracting what you don't want into your life, that's when the healing work really begins.

Healing through Dreams

During the day, notice when that mindset strikes. Don't criticize or judge it, just notice it and choose to release the thoughts and feelings that have created it. Let them all go.

Then replace those limiting thoughts and feelings with thoughts and feelings about what you actually want to attract into your life. Expect good things to come your way.

Ask your dreams to reflect your progress back to you.

When you start dreaming about the life you want, you will know your chances of manifesting it are closer than ever.

Repeat this process every time you want to bring more healing and joy into your life.

CREATIVITY

There are stacks of examples of dreams inspiring innovations, inventions and scientific breakthroughs. Einstein, for instance, was a big dreamer, with many of his scientific breakthroughs, such as the speed of light and the theory of relativity, being inspired by his dreams.

Dreams really can ignite your inner artist too. Surrealist painter Salvador Dalí described his celebrated artwork as 'hand-painted photographs of my dreams'. Should you ever suffer from writer's or creative block, grab your dream journal and read your last dream. It will remove that block right away.

Stephen King says he uses his dreams 'in the same way you would use a mirror to look at the back of your head'. He believes the purpose of dreams is to help people understand the nature of their problems, or sometimes to offer answers to those problems in symbolic language. Many of his own novels are based on his night visions.

If you are preoccupied with a problem in waking life or experiencing a creative block, asking your dreaming mind for help can bring a revelation and sometimes even a solution. Elias Howe said that he got his idea for the sewing machine from a dream in which he was captured by cannibals dancing around a fire. They had spears with tiny holes in and the up and down movement of the spears and the holes gave him the idea for passing a thread through the tip of the needle.

Physicist Niels Bohr dreamed he was sitting on the sun and all the planets were spinning around him on threads. This dream lingered with him and eventually became the Eureka moment that led to the development of the Bohr model of the atom.

John Newton, a slave trader and the composer of the song 'Amazing Grace', became an abolitionist after a dream of Europe being consumed by a raging fire.

You never know what will be the result of your next dream. Perhaps it will become a book, or a movie, or a game (many movie directors and game designers plunder their dreams for content), or a perfume, or a business idea. But whether your next dream changes the world or not, if it changes your life for the better, that is just as valuable, as we are all interconnected and one person healing their life lights a candle that can illuminate all those who cross their path.

LUCID DREAMS

Asking your dreams for help before you go to sleep is a potent way to investigate and resolve your personal growth roadblocks, but you can, if you have the time and discipline, take this a step further and enter the world of lucid dreaming.

Lucid dreaming is being aware you are dreaming when you are dreaming. It gets a lot of attention nowadays and is the most researched aspect of dreaming. I'm going to reference the Senoi Temiar tribe of Malaysia here, because they place lucid dreaming centre-stage in their lives. They are a gentle and peaceful people who appear to be free of depression and crime. Could their devotion to lucid dreaming be the reason?

From an early age, Temiar children are encouraged to share their dreams with the rest of the tribe and taught techniques to influence their dreams. If they dream of being attacked by a wild animal, they are taught how to re-enter that dream in the lucid dreaming state to face and defeat that predator. The idea is that being brave in their dreams will translate into their waking lives – a kind of threat rehearsal or role-play – and potentially save their lives.

Temiar teenagers don't seem to report nightmares, because they have been taught to use lucid dream skills to overcome their fears in a dream. They are encouraged to seek out positive symbols and settings too, as it is believed that a positive dream inspires a positive day. Taking charge of their dreams helps them feel confident and happy in their waking lives.

There remains some debate about the quality of the research done on the Temiar tribe, but even so there is much we can learn from their belief that directing your dreams can help you direct your life.

Lucid dreaming has been shown to ease symptoms of PTSD in veterans, according to a study by the Institute of Noetic Sciences (IONS) and lucid dreaming expert Charlie Morley, and to be a helpful tool for athletes and musicians to practise skills while they are sleeping. You may think this sounds far-fetched, but your brain doesn't actually know the difference between dreaming and the waking state, so if you rehearse or practise or role-play in a dream, you are reinforcing the pathways in your brain that have been created to help you learn or prepare for something in your waking life.

I cover lucid dreaming in depth and the techniques used to induce it in *How to Catch a Dream*. The issue is that some of these techniques disrupt your sleep, which is not recommended for your holistic well-being and therefore your dream work.

The best way to increase your chances of having a lucid dream is to induce it naturally by doubling down on your dream recall and following all the decoding advice in this book. The more seriously you take your dreams, the more likely you are to have those rare lucid ones.

But please don't worry if they don't happen. It takes a lot of time and dedication to master the art of lucid dreaming, and although it can offer incredible possibilities, it is really just another way to dream. So, please don't get caught up with chasing this elusive state. In my opinion, the symbolic dreams you have night after night have far greater self-help potential, because they are constantly there for you, tirelessly offering support and guidance.

My advice is: just as you would in waking life, invest your time and energy in what's always there for you, rather than fly-by-nights.

LET'S GET LIMINAL

I'd like to conclude this night school with another shout-out for the transformative power of those suggestible and intensely creative liminal states between waking and sleeping and sleeping and waking.

Just as you may be able to have some influence over the kind of dreams you have, so you can also utilize the transitional periods between wakefulness and sleep to become aware of surreal or out-there ideas that pop into your brain on their own. This is known as hypnagogic or liminal dreaming.

While you won't be able to control your dreams during this state, you can harness the sensational creativity that can come out of them – as long as you wake yourself up to remember it and don't fall into a deep sleep. Remember they happen every night when you go to sleep and wake up, but you may not be aware of them or want to wake up and write down what happens in them.

The best-known way to wake yourself up during hypnagogia is to close your eyes and doze off sitting upright in a comfortable chair while holding something in an outstretched hand that's resting on the side of the chair – something that won't break when dropped, such as a metal spoon, and will make a noise when it hits the floor. That way, when you drop off to sleep, you'll drop the object, and the noise of it falling will snap you out of your hypnagogic state, hopefully remembering the ideas that came to you while you were in it.

Taking a mid-afternoon nap is the optimum way to become more aware of the liminal states. Napping has been shown to be a natural concentration and creativity booster, and the reason is that your dreaming mind senses, due to daylight clues, that this isn't going to be a full-blown sleep, so fast-forwards you to the edges of REM sleep, which is crucial for your brain power and holistic well-being.

Taking a regular afternoon nap may in fact be one of the best ways to stimulate dream recall and also to boost your levels of mental alertness. Around 20 to 30-minute naps are optimum, so if your schedule permits, include a mid-afternoon nap in your day. You have nothing to lose and only increased well-being and dream inspiration to gain.

And if taking a nap isn't for you, taking five or ten minutes out of your day to sit quietly and simply let your mind wander or daydream is another way to dream, the only difference being that you are wide awake and fully in control of the direction of that dream.

DÉJÀ RÊVÉ

Congratulations – you have almost completed your night school.

Stop now and ask yourself if you've started to notice aspects of your dreams – symbols, themes, colours, sounds or feelings – in your waking life. If you haven't, I strongly urge you to start seeking out aspects of your dreams every day in your waking life. For example, if you dream of a rose, buy yourself a bunch the next day, or if you dream of a fictional character, read the book that they are in, and so on. Just be sensible and make sure you seek out aspects that are safe and will harm no one.

You'll notice that in your dream journal template I encourage you to keep a record of when and how you encounter elements from your dreams in your waking life. But don't leave that to chance, start making it happen by proactively seeking them out. In time this should become a key part of your dream work, because the more you do it, the more likely it will be that over time your dream symbols will start appearing in your waking life in *déjà-rêvé* moments.

When this happens, stop and reflect in awe on the wisdom of your dreaming mind. As mentioned earlier, the symbol is likely to be trivial, but it indicates that this is *the* moment for you to stop and reflect on the current direction of your life. If you don't like that direction or don't feel good about it, your *déjà rêvé* is a reminder that there is so much more to you and your life than meets the eye and you always have a *choice*.

Déjà rêvé is more than coincidence. According to Jung, it is synchronicity, which is a meaningful coincidence, a sign that you are awakening from the inside out. It is also a potent manifesting sign, reinforcing to you that it isn't what you dream but how you respond to your dreams that is key to your healing and growth.

You are the creator of your own dreams, as they reflect your unconscious beliefs about yourself. If you don't like your dreams and how they make you feel, you can change that right here, right now, by changing your beliefs. The power is in you in this moment *now*. Dreams teach you to become aware of your choices and how they – not external forces – determine how satisfied you feel. And when your beliefs change, not only do your dreams become more empowering and constantly updated with exciting new themes, but your waking life transforms into something better. You are healing, or should I say returning to your true nature, from the inside out, and when you do, you start to attract magic into your life.

And it all starts with a memory of a dream and the awareness that it is never, *ever* 'just' a dream!

CONCLUSION
YOU ARE A DREAM

Night light:
What you think you create.
What you feel you attract.
What you dream you become.
Your future is always looking back at you
in your dreams.

As this book draws to a close, don't think of this as the end of your dream adventure but the entry point. To reference the timeless wisdom of T.S. Eliot, to reach the end is to find yourself at the beginning again, but knowing yourself for the very first time. That is because every dream recalled is a return to wholeness, your true self, but not a circle or loop back, a spiral where you see yourself from ever-higher perspectives.

All those dreams point to the same inescapable conclusion: you can't find meaning outside yourself. It can't be found in the material stuff, the approval of other people and the acquisition of things. The only way is in – you need to voyage deep into your own inner space.

This isn't to say the material is irrelevant, far from it. The material world and all the wonders in it offer an opportunity to be challenged and to learn and grow, and the meaning of our lives is found in learning and growing. But the material world is not and never will be what truly defines you. What defines you is your inner world, the world you get up close and personal with every night in your dreams.

And if you believe in the possibility of life after death, your inner world – your consciousness, your heart – is the part of you that may go on.

Until then, your dreams will always be there for you, like guardian angels watching over you each night, offering endless inner lights to guide you back to your loving centre or source, which is your heart. Remember your dream cure mantra: all the meaning, all the healing and all the love you need can be found alive and kicking within your own dreams.

TIME FLIES BY

In the words of physicist Niels Bohr, 'Everything we call real is made of things that cannot be regarded as real.' Dreams can feel incredibly real and we have all woken up in the morning and taken a few moments to recognize that whatever we just experienced happened in the dream state and not the waking world.

Elderly people often say that the more the years fly by, the more they lose track of time and their lives start to feel like a living dream. Past, present and future begin to merge and waking life can sometimes feel as surreal and fragmented as a dream.

When you start to tune into the healing potential of your dreams, you may also start to feel more timeless as you discover an inner awareness that may have been absent before. This shift happens because your dreams take you to an unseen place where feelings are the currency and everything you thought you knew about this life and everything you thought was important is turned on its head. Dreams encourage you to take a leap of faith beyond logic, and whenever you do that, creativity is born and real magic bursts forth. You may also find that you start to recall more dreams happening within dreams. This is always exciting as it suggests deeper inner exploration.

If you don't think you are a creative force, your dreams will show you that the force is alive within you. If you don't think you are spiritually inclined, they will show you that you are deep beyond measure. They connect you to your inner artist, healer and shaman, to your very essence, which is always curious, always brainstorming and always seeking meaning beneath the surface.

The next time you recall a dream and one of its symbols, here's another head-scratching question to ask yourself: Are you a human dreaming you are that symbol or is that symbol dreaming you are a human?

Dreams reflect who you really are. What if when you dream, you are actually reconnecting with what is real, with your true essence, and visiting the home of your soul? Up to 90 per cent of what we think we experience is unseen, and it is impossible to describe the human experience in purely factual or material terms without reference to forces that are unseen. And real meaning can only ever be found in what is unseen. To quote Helen Keller, 'The best things in life are unseen. That is why we close our eyes when we cry, kiss and dream.'

What if the external material world is the dream and the only path to happiness, the only reality, is within your dreams?

YOUR DREAM ORACLE IMPERATIVE

The term 'dream oracle' is a much misunderstood one and I don't want you to use it lightly, but if you have followed the guidance in this book and are paying close attention to your dreams, *congratulations*. You are graduating from night school and have my full permission to call yourself your own dream oracle.

And now, with the basic principles of dream work secure in your mind, heart and soul, you may want to take another giant leap of faith and use your newfound insight to not just heal and empower yourself, but to help heal and empower others. Indeed, if you are on track with your dream work, this is what you will instinctively feel called to do. You will want to share the healing power of what you know with others. Dream work increases empathy, because you know that we are all dreaming beings.

Many people still don't know how to decode their dreams, however, so I urge you to become a light for others in dark places. Ask them about their dreams. Don't overwhelm them, but if they are receptive, offer a few pointers to help them interpret their dreams for themselves. Tell them their dreams are their inner therapist. If they share a dream with you, remember the golden rule that you must apply both to your own dreams and to those you decode for others: *always* offer a positive and uplifting interpretation. A dream interpretation that leaves the dreamer feeling anxious is not the correct interpretation.

Remember, too, that when people share a dream with you, even though they don't realize it, they are actually sharing a piece of their soul. Treat their dreams with reverence and respect. Keep them private. Unless I am given permission to share, that is what I have always done when people message me their dreams to decipher, and I will continue to do so.

Should you be in a position to share your newfound illumination with loved ones or on your social media or at school or in the workplace, you'll find that in the majority of cases you won't be met with resistance or disapproval. I've spent the last few decades mainstreaming the self-help potential of dream work and removing fear of it in the process with national viewer call-ins on TV and radio. I'm over the moon to say that the response has been reassuringly positive. People love talking about their dreams. It is a brilliant ice-breaker.

Everyone, including those who are highly sceptical and rational, will have had a dream that they want to understand. Help them understand it. A great way to do that is to interpret it for them as if it were yours and then ask them to reflect on the feelings that interpretation inspires in them.

Be the dream you want to see in the world.

My dream is to one day see the basic tools of dream work taught at primary schools in the same way that parents and elders of the Senoi Temiar and Pirahã teach their young children. With rates of depression and anxiety soaring in young people today, the more children are encouraged to lose their fear of their own intuition and creativity and to trust in their dreams and discover within themselves the power to shine brightly, however dark the world around them can seem, the better. I also anticipate a time when dream work is taught in prisons, to help offenders understand the motives for their actions and come to terms with their shadow.

Dream work can also find a natural home in doctors' surgeries, hospices and hospitals to help patients understand the mind–body connection in the healing process. And dream work should be a part of any anger-management programme, and a mainstay of grief counsellors and therapists.

DREAMING WITH OTHERS

There will be times in your dream work when you get stuck, and when this happens, you may want to share a dream with someone you trust. Sometimes just telling someone else about a dream can spark an insight.

And if you feel comfortable sharing your dreams, and others feel safe sharing their dreams with you, then you may want to take your dream oracle credentials to their inevitable conclusion and consider dreaming *on behalf of* others. Let them give you a question and then dream on it on their behalf.

If you have been doing the exercises and understand the information in this book, you are fully qualified to become a dream oracle.

When you share your dream symbols with the person you are dreaming for, simply narrate them and then encourage the person to come to their own conclusions. This may sound very far out, but it can be an incredibly healing experience for them and also for you. It can also deepen your own understanding of dreams, and that is the wonder of dream work.

You need never be bored. There is always more to learn, more to uncover.

For now, revisit the dream power points on page 4 and imprint them on your mind and heart.

IT'S YOUR DREAM

At the end of the night, I hope this book will have made it abundantly clear that dream decoding isn't for the therapist, or even the dream specialist, or something you look up in a book or online. It is a tool for personal growth and manifestation that you can use repeatedly to deepen your self-knowledge and improve your chances of attracting success and happiness into your life.

You are going to dream anyway, so you might as well make the best of your dreams. And in the process of meeting, catching and befriending your night visions, I promise you your life will never be the same again. Knowing what your dreams mean can heal your life. And it will heal it in the best possible sense, by reminding you that you don't actually need to be healed, as this suggests sickness and lack. It will remind you that whatever happens in your waking life, everything is a lesson or blessing. All you truly need is to remember and trust in your own inner power, your own dreams, which have always been there for you. You just need to clear what obscures them, and more often than not, what obscures them is your own lack of faith in them.

Satisfaction is going to bed each night with your soul at peace, ready to incubate incredible dreams.

Joy is starting your day with gratitude and dreams saturating your mind.

You will know when you have become a full-blown dream oracle, because the next time you wake up with the words, 'I have a dream,' it will become a source of the greatest joy, often eclipsing what is happening externally in your life. This is because waking up with a dream on your mind and gratitude in your heart is proof that your brain is awake, your inner world is on fire and you are truly, madly, deeply *alive*.

There is no longer any disconnection or disassociation between your waking and dream life and no more fear of your unconscious depths, even if what is revealed in your dreams is shocking or alarming, because instead of anxiety you only feel excitement about the surprising personal insights and deep revelations about the wonder of you that are to come. You don't just have a 'dream' anymore. You are now living, and flying in the direction of, your dreams.

RESOURCES

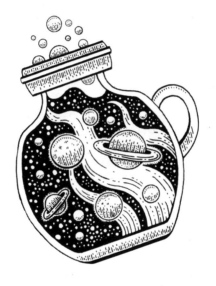

YOUR DREAM CURE JOURNAL TEMPLATES

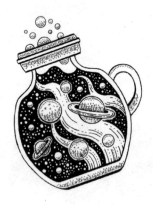

Based on the dream cure principles in this book, I encourage you to follow the 20:20 Night Vision Template below, using a blank sheet of paper (A4 size is ideal), for a minimum of 20 days.

Up until your 21st dream, simply enjoy recalling and writing down your dreams. If you go through a period of no recall, wait until a dream memory comes. It is important you hit the 20th dream mark *before* you begin your dream journal and your dream decoding in earnest.

YOUR 20:20 NIGHT VISION TEMPLATE

YOUR MORNING DREAM TIME
(2 TO 3 MINUTES)

Date:

Feeling on waking:

Key words/symbols recalled on waking:

Dream theme(s) identified:

Dream space:
[This space is for you to draw images from your dream, give your dream a title or anything else you would like to record from your night of dreaming.]

When you reach Dream 21, it's time to invest in a blank notebook and follow the Dream Journal Template overleaf. I suggest you make sure there is ample space for you to write, because once you start recording your dreams, trust me, those recollections will flow.

YOUR DREAM JOURNAL TEMPLATE

Let the dream decoding begin!

[Left-hand page in your dream journal]
YOUR MORNING DREAM TIME
(2 TO 3 MINUTES)

Date:

Feeling on waking:

Key words/symbols recalled on waking:

Dream theme(s) identified:

Any recurring theme(s):

Dream space:
[This space is for you to draw images from your dream, give your dream a title or anything else you would like to record from your night of dreaming.]

Instant associations:

Any symbols recalled later in the day:

[Right-hand page]
YOUR EVENING DREAM TIME
(MINIMUM 5 MINUTES)

Key events that took place during the day:

Déjà rêvé moments in the day when you 'met' or actively
sought out elements of your dream:

Any possible literal considerations to rule out:

Select up to three symbols/themes from the previous
night's dream and brainstorm associations:

Symbol 1:
Associations:

Symbol 2:
Associations:

Symbol 3:
Associations:

Connections between dream and waking life:
Question(s) to ask your dream:

Positive interpretation of the dream:
Positive action or mindset change inspired by the dream:

Dreamscaping intention/request on sleeping:

INDEX OF
DREAM THEMES

accidents, 109, 134, 135

acting, 142

action, 135–6

adventure *see* action

affairs *see* cheating; sex and erotica

afterlife communication, 221–3

Air (element) *see* birds; elements

airport, 146

ambition, 136–7

amphibians, 137

anger, 84, 150, 158, 199, 206

animals, 137–9

ants *see* insects

anus, 83

anxiety, 18, 30, 37, 49, 63, 64, 68, 94, 96, 98, 99, 116, 122, 128, 129, 131, 158, 166, 170, 194, 201, 215, 239, 255, 258; *see also* fear

archetypes, 139–42

arms, 83

artistic endeavours, 142–3

astrology *see* magic

attack *see* conflict; disaster; violence; *also* animals; fear

audience, 142–3; *see also* artistic endeavours

autumn, 174

avalanche *see* disasters

baby, 101–2, 128, 141, 144; *see also* birth; pregnancy

back, 83

badger, 138

balloon *see* elements (Air)

bees *see* insects

beige, 150

bike *see* travel

birds, 143–4

birth, 144; *see also* baby; pregnancy

black, 150

blood, 189

blue, 150

body, 23, 145
    parts, 82–3

bones, 189

bread, 161

breasts, 83

breathing *see* elements (Air)

bridge, 147
brown, 150
building, 145–6
burglar, 164
burial, 210

calendar *see* time
car crash, 215; *see also* out-of-control
    car
castle, 146
celebrity, 59, 124–5, 177, 212
challenges, 41–7
change, 42, 146–7, 153, 155, 201, 211,
    212, 219, 239, 240, 244, 249; *see also*
    disaster
chased, 84–5
cheating, 85–6; *see also* sex and
    erotica
chess, 168
chest, 83, 204
chewing gum, 86–7
childhood, 61, 79, 99, 121–3, 147, 164,
    168, 171, 177, 204, 207, 212
children, 147–8
    unborn, 223–4
church, 36, 146
circle, 188
climbing, 148
clock *see* time
clothes, 148–9; *see also* nudity
colours, 149–51
communication, 151, 221–3
computers *see* media and technology
conflict, 151–2

cooking *see* food and drink
corpse, burying, 124
court, 146
crime, 194, 245
crowd *see* gatherings
crystals *see* jewellery; *also* magic

daisies, 161
dancing *see* action
death and dying, 87, 210–13
deformity, 189
departed loved ones, 131, 161, 221–3;
    see also flowers,
destruction *see* conflict; *also* disaster
detective, 178
disappointment, 129
disaster, 152–5, 214
disguise, 136
doctor, 189
dove *see* love
dragons *see* surrealism
drinking *see* food and drink
drowning, 23, 87–9, 123, 152, 198, 213

ears, 83
Earth (element), 155–6
eating *see* food and drink
e-mail, 151
elements, 155–6
elevation *see* climbing
end-of-the-world scenarios, 153–4
everyday items, 157
examinations, 89–90
eyes, 83, 242

factory, 146

failure, 89–90, 126, 129, 239;
  see also examinations;
  unpreparedness

fairies see surrealism

falling, 90–2; see also elements (Air)

familiar people or surroundings,
  125–6

familiar tasks becoming impossible,
  125–6

family, 157–8; see also people

famous people, 124

fasting see food and drink

father, 158

fear, 158–9; see also anxiety; chased;
  disasters; threat

feet, 83

fictional characters, 59, 176, 248

field, 174

finding, 192–3

fingers, 83

fire, 93–4; see also elements

fish, 150

floating, 156

flowers, 160–1

flying, 94–5; see also elements
  (Air); joy; missed flight or
  train; travel

food and drink, 161

foreign country, 162

forest, 173–4

forest fire see disasters

fox, 138

frustration, 169–70

gambling, 168

games, 44–5, 244; see also leisure
  pursuits

gatherings, 162–3

gemstones, 166; see also jewellery

genitals, 83; see also sex and erotica

gifts, 163

gold (colour), 111, 150, 173

goodbyes, 147

gorging see food and drink

grass see elements (Earth); also nature

green, 150

grey, 150

groups see gatherings

hair, 83
  falling out, 95–6

hand, 130–1

hare, 138

hat, 149

head, 83

health, 31, 40–1, 44, 82, 106, 145, 189

heart, 34, 50, 63, 83, 90, 106, 215, 225;
  see also love

hobbies see leisure activities

holidays, 163

home, 164–5; see also property damage

horror, 217

hospital, 189, 256

hotel, 146

injury, 213

insects, 165

internet, the, see media and technology,

jewellery, 166; *see also* gemstones

joy, 166–7

jumping *see* action

killing *see* conflict; *also* murder

labyrinth, 147

lake, 174

language, 45; *see also* foreign country; speech

late, 96–7

leisure activities, 167–8

legs, 83

letters of the alphabet, 169

library, 146

lighthouse, 146

location, 182–3

loss, 97–8

lost, 62, 97–8, 169–70, 179, 181

lottery win, 92, 160, 167, 172

love, 4, 22, 170

lovers, 183–8

    former, 184

    unknown, 184

    vanishing, 187

luggage, 163

lungs, 69, 83

magic, 128, 138, 170–1, 191; *see also* surrealism

magpie, 143

maze, 147

media, 171–2; *see also* communication; social media

medicine, 189

microwave, 157

mirror, 75, 208–9, 241, 242

missed flight or train, 126

money, 172–3

monsters, 84, 122, 123, 141

moon *see* space

mother, 9, 105, 139, 173

motion *see* travel

mountain, 223

mouth *see* chewing gum; *also* food and drink

movie, 112, 142, 168, 176, 198, 204, 217

mud *see* elements (Earth); *also* nature

murder, 140, 211, 233

museum, 146

music, 46–7, 113, 143

nature, 74, 113, 150, 173–4

neck, 83

nightwear, 148–9

nose, 83

nudity, 98–100; *see also* clothes

numbers, 174–5

nun, 176

obstacles, 129, 192–3, 200

orange (colour), 150

out-of-control vehicle, 100, 215

panic, 88, 111, 159

paralysis, 214

party *see* gatherings

past lives, 224

people, 175–8
  family, 157–8
  famous, 124–5, 176, 177
  from your past, 177
phone, 39, 65, 130, 151, 171–2, 174; *see also* communication
photographs *see* time
pink, 150
plane crash, 154
planets *see* space
plants, 174; *see also* flowers
play (drama), 168; *see also* artistic endeavours
poison, 152
position (of dreamer), 62–3
precognition, 182
pregnancy, 101–2, 128, 223; *see also* baby; birth
prison, 146, 256
prize, 178
problem, 178–80
property damage, 215
purple, 150

racing *see* action
radio, 172
railway station, 146
red, 150
rejection, 128, 129, 200, 238
religion, 180
reptiles *see* amphibians
rest-room, 102
river, 174
romance *see* love; sex and erotica

roses, 161
running *see* action; travel; *also* chased

'saved the day', 201–2
school, 74–5, 110, 122, 127, 147, 180–1
sea, 150
secret room, 159
servant, 176
setting, 182
sex and erotica, 183–8
shaman *see* magic
siblings, 122, 158, 225, 240
sickness, 189
silver (colour), 151
sinking ship, 154
skin, 83
snakes, 102–3, 185, 227
social media, 15, 99, 171, 172, 255; *see also* nudity; media and technology
soil *see* elements (Earth); *also* nature
soldier, 176
sorcerer *see* magic
space, 190
speech, 190; *see also* language
spell *see* magic
spider, 104–5, 165
sport *see* leisure activities
spring (season), 174
square, 188
stage, 125, 142
star *see* shapes; *also* space
stomach, 63, 83
storm *see* drowning; elements (Air, Water); *also* thunderstorm

stranger, 84, 86, 141, 175, 178, 187, 212

summer, 174, 182

sun *see* space

superhero powers, 123, 136–7, 139, 167; *see also* joy

surrealism, 190–1, 243

swimming *see* elements (Water)

Tarot *see* magic

teachers, 19, 89, 122, 178, 180

technology, 171–2

teeth falling out, 106–7

telepathy, 182, 226

television, 172

threat *see* chased; conflict; crime; violence; *also* snakes

throat, 83

thunderstorm, 111–12, 182

time, 48, 191; *see also* clock; numbers

tornado *see* disasters; drowning

toys, 122, 168

traffic lights, 157

travel, 62, 192–3; *see also* foreign country; missed flight or train; out-of-control car

treasure, 92–3, 160, 172–3

trees *see* elements (Earth); *also* nature

triangle (shape), 188

tsunami *see* disasters; drowning

unicorns *see* surrealism

unpreparedness, 90, 125, 126, 127, 181, 200; *see also* examinations; late; school

valuables, 98, 160

violence, 193–4; *see also* conflict

volcano *see* disasters

walking *see* travel

warfare *see* conflict

washing, 156

watch *see* time

water *see* elements (Water); *also* drowning

weapon *see* conflict; violence

weather *see* setting

wedding *see* gatherings

whale, 160

white, 151

windows, 159

winter, 174

witch *see* magic

work, 194–5
    career-ending blunder, 194–5
    different career, 195

world conspiring against you, 199–201, 202

writing, 195

yellow, 151

SUGGESTED READING, LISTENING, WATCHING, VISITING

READING
Books

Theresa Cheung, *Dream Dictionary A to Z* (HarperElement, 2004, 2009; Thorsons, 2019)

Sigmund Freud, *The Interpretation of Dreams* (Franz Deuticke, 1899; Macmillan, 1913; Wordsworth Editions, 1997)

C.G. Jung, *Memories, Dreams, Reflections* (Exlibris, 1962; Pantheon Books, 1963; Fontana, 1995)

Guy Leschziner, *The Nocturnal Brain* (Simon & Schuster, 2019)

Frederick S. Perls, *Gestalt Therapy Verbatim* (The Gestalt Journal Press, 2013)

Matthew Walker, *Why We Sleep* (Penguin, 2018)

Articles

https://greatergood.berkeley.edu/article/item/why_your_brain
   _needs_to_dream

https://www.ncbi.nlm.nih.gov/pmc/articles/PMC6428732/

http://nectar.northampton.ac.uk/8241/

https://noetic.org/research/extraordinary-experiences-and
-performance-on-psi-tasks-during-and-after-meditation
-classes-and-retreats/

https://nyaspubs.onlinelibrary.wiley.com/doi/abs/10.1111/nyas
.13447

https://psycnet.apa.org/doiLanding?doi=10.1037%2Ftrm0000456

https://www.sciencedaily.com/releases/2023/08/230828162332.htm

https://www.sleepfoundation.org/dreams

https://www.theguardian.com/lifeandstyle/2023/sep/20/the-sleep
-secret-how-lucid-dreams-can-make-us-fitter-more-creative
-and-less-anxious

https://time.com/4970767/rem-sleep-dreams-health/

LISTENING

White Shores, hosted by Theresa Cheung, is an audio-only podcast
on all free podcast platforms. The following *White Shores*
episodes are all dream themed:

Season 4, Ep. 12: 'Behind your Eyes' with Dr Clare Johnson

Season 6, Ep. 4: 'Lottery Dreams' with Tim Schultz

Season 6, Ep. 7: 'Your Presence, Dear' with Gary Lachman

Season 6, Ep. 9: 'True Dream Circle' with Charlie Morley

Season 6, Ep. 10: 'Pure Nonsense' with Dr Julia Mossbridge and
Brooks Palmer

Season 6, Ep. 12: 'Meet Dr Sleep' with Bawa and Dinesch

Season 6, Ep. 13: 'Diving Deep into your Dreams' with Dr Clare
Johnson

Season 6, Ep. 15: 'Psychic Dreams' with Loyd Auberach

Season 6, Ep. 19: 'Messages from the Deep' with Lauri Loewenberg

Season 6, Ep. 20: 'Your Time Loops' with Eric Wargo

Season 6, Ep. 25: 'An Endless Dream Talk'

Season 6, Ep. 31: 'World Dream Day'

Season 6, Ep. 32: 'Your Dream Notes'

Season 6, Ep. 41: 'Heads Up Dreaming' with Prof. Carlyle Smith

Season 7 Ep. 2: 'What Dreams May Come' with Brian Smith

Season 7, Ep. 29: 'Vibes, Dreams and Tears' with Dr Garret Yount

Season 8, Ep. 1: 'What Dreams Have Come' with Stephen Simon

Season 8, Ep. 4: 'Believe Your Dream' with Athena Laz

Season 8, Ep. 5: 'Your Night Vision' with Lauri Loewenberg

Season 8, Ep. 6: 'Your Unforgettable Dream' with Dr Clare Johnson

Season 8, Ep. 9: 'Death is But a Dream' with Sandra Champlain

In your Dreamzz audio-only podcast hosted by Alex Morgan and featuring Theresa Cheung

WATCHING
Movies

The Wizard of Oz (1939)

What Dreams May Come (1998)

Inception (2010)

Dune (2021)

Slumberland (2022)

TV series

Sandman (2022)

VISITING

Institute of Noetic Sciences (IONS): https://noetic.org

International Association for the Study of Dreams (IASD): www.asdreams.org

The Institute for Dream Studies (IDS): https://institutefordream studies.org

ACKNOWLEDGEMENTS

Sincere gratitude to my publishers, HarperCollins, for their faith in my dream work, to my editor, Lydia Good, for her kindness, wisdom and support, to my copy-editor, Lizzie Henry, for her insight and brilliant fine-tuning, and to everyone involved in the production of this book.

I would also like to thank all the scientists and dream researchers I have worked with along the way and all the 'powered by dreams' experts I have interviewed on my *White Shores* podcast. Special thanks to Gail Torr from Galaxy Media for being a dream to work with.

Heartfelt thanks also to my family. I could not have written this book without your love and my little dog, Arnie, being by my side.

Most important of all are my readers and listeners. You are the stuff that dreams are made of and a constant source of illumination to me. Thank you from my heart and soul.

ABOUT THE AUTHOR

Theresa Cheung is a *Sunday Times* bestselling dreams author.

She has a degree from King's College, Cambridge, and is the author of numerous titles which have been translated into over 40 languages, including *The Dream Dictionary from A to Z* (HarperCollins), *How to Catch a Dream* (HarperCollins), *Empower Your Inner Psychic* (HarperCollins) and *The Dream Decoder Card Pack* and *Dream Rituals Oracle Card Pack* (Hachette).

Theresa works closely with scientists researching consciousness and dreams and has contributed features about dreams to national and international newspapers and magazines, including *Bustle*, *Vice*, *Cosmopolitan*, *Good Housekeeping*, *InStyle*, *Red*, *Grazia*, *Heat*, *Metro*, *Glamour* and many more. She has been interviewed by Claudia Winkleman on BBC Radio 2, Nicky Campbell on BBC Radio 5 Live, Roman Kemp on Capital Radio, Regina Meredith on Gaia TV, George Noory on Coast to Coast AM, Piers Morgan on ITV, Terrence Lee on Fox News, Chicago, and by other leading media outlets, including KTLA, Today Extra, Channel 4 and local BBC Radio. The subject of a night poet episode on Nicky Campbell's BBC Sounds 5 Live podcast, *Different*, and a frequent dream-decoding guest on ITV's *This Morning*, Theresa has hosted numerous national dream call-ins live on TV and decoded dreams for many celebrities and influencers. She has given dream-decoding talks and webinars to leading companies and brands, such as Action Coach, Anthropologie, Beauty Bay, Dynavision, Immediate Media, Shiseido and the Hearst magazine group. She also hosts her own popular podcast, *White Shores*.

CONTACT THERESA, QUEEN OF DREAMS

You can message, ask questions, share your dreams with and follow Theresa on Instagram @thetheresacheung and via her Facebook and X author pages, and learn more about her dream work at www.theresacheung.com.

Every great dream begins with a dreamer. Always remember you have within you the strength, the patience, and the passion to reach for the stars, to change your world.

Harriet Tubman